Joel Macht

The Medicalization of America's Schools

Challenging the Concept of Educational Disabilities

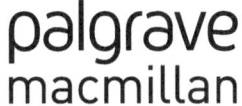

Joel Macht
Davidson, North Carolina, USA

Joel Macht
Davidson, North Carolina, USA

ISBN 978-3-319-62973-5   ISBN 978-3-319-62974-2 (eBook)
DOI 10.1007/978-3-319-62974-2

Library of Congress Control Number: 2017949872

© The Editor(s) (if applicable) and The Author(s) 2017
This work is subject to copyright. All rights are solely and exclusively licensed by the Publisher, whether the whole or part of the material is concerned, specifically the rights of translation, reprinting, reuse of illustrations, recitation, broadcasting, reproduction on microfilms or in any other physical way, and transmission or information storage and retrieval, electronic adaptation, computer software, or by similar or dissimilar methodology now known or hereafter developed.
The use of general descriptive names, registered names, trademarks, service marks, etc. in this publication does not imply, even in the absence of a specific statement, that such names are exempt from the relevant protective laws and regulations and therefore free for general use.
The publisher, the authors and the editors are safe to assume that the advice and information in this book are believed to be true and accurate at the date of publication. Neither the publisher nor the authors or the editors give a warranty, express or implied, with respect to the material contained herein or for any errors or omissions that may have been made. The publisher remains neutral with regard to jurisdictional claims in published maps and institutional affiliations.

Cover design by Ran Shauli

Printed on acid-free paper

This Palgrave Macmillan imprint is published by Springer Nature
The registered company is Springer International Publishing AG
The registered company address is: Gewerbestrasse 11, 6330 Cham, Switzerland

ACKNOWLEDGMENTS

Thanks to Lee, Nancy, Jack, and Jon, the children at the Valley of the Sun, those at SEMBCS, those at Davidson Community, those I've met over these many years, and always my own, all my mentors.

And the Dragon, who with effort will be slayed.

CONTENTS

LIST OF BOXES

CHAPTER 1

From Educational Differences to Educational Disabilities

I made my way through grade school and high school in the 1950s and never once met face-to-face any classmate with more obvious challenges than a kid negotiating a crowded school wearing a sling to support a broken arm. If children who fared worse than my friends or me existed, I never knew about them, nor who they were, nor where they lived.

As a boy in the mid-1940s, I had my own scare with polio, but the high fever melted away without any trace of what annually frightened a large segment of the US population. I was too young to have understood what might have happened had the poliovirus established itself. Had I the words in those carefree days, I'd have described life as fair, decent, and thoroughly equitable. I'd have to wait until my 20s before my naiveté was ripped away.

Behavioral Psychology Laboratory; Educational Practices

It was the late summer of 1966. I attended Arizona State University, the doctoral program in psychology. Knowing few specifics of the recommended course, I drove into the desert to the psychology department's behavioral laboratory attached to a state-operated residential facility for children. The term "residential" had no special meaning, and I'd have done poorly on any quiz that asked me to describe who I expected to

© The Author(s) 2017
J. Macht, *The Medicalization of America's Schools*,
DOI 10.1007/978-3-319-62974-2_1

find living at the state's center. Equally eager and anxious, I parked on my side of an encapsulating linked fence built high enough to keep outside out and inside in. Standing under a spacious sky, I glanced at the residential center's bleak and vacant landscape. The effect was unsettling. I had expected groups of children running about, laughing, playing games, a park with swings and seesaws and a nearby duck pond.

They saw me first. Two of them, buddies standing side by side. Short-statured, they gawked at me, their faces flat and broad, their eyes oddly shaped, their mouths drooped lazily, their tongues wide and large and protruding. I judged they were eight or nine years old, with no assurance that my guess was close.

Unsettled by their look, I managed my best smile, told the boys my name and asked them theirs. Staring back, they remained silent. I thought they were waiting for me to say more. For someone who was an inveterate yapper, I was straightaway tongue tied, grateful the boys didn't ask me what I was doing on their property.

One stretched his fingers toward me through the fence, a universal invitation. When I touched his fingers, he smiled. "Thank you," I said with a sigh of relief. At once I wanted to be on their side of the fence. They were just kids—like all kids—with differences. Not liking the fence, or the boys' captive place behind it, I made small talk mostly to relieve my persisting unease.

I looked about and realized this was their home, day and night. It seemed a thoroughly inhospitable setting, desolate and disconnected, as if designed intentionally to keep itself out of sight, not unlike an embarrassing generational relic you'd hide from neighbors. I couldn't help thinking that it was not a proper place anyone should call "home." I looked at the boys. Was that what this off-campus course was all about? These youngsters? Someone's children? I wondered what I could do for them, something that might better their lives. Nothing came to mind, my earlier graduate training without any connection. That didn't sit well. With little confidence, I wished the boys a good day and headed toward a flat-roofed cinderblock building, my steps without their characteristic bounce.

I entered the behavior lab that would become my home for nearly three years. Within days, I switched programs to the Educational Psychology department to be mentored by one of its professors who co-directed the laboratory. Nothing about me would ever be the same.

The class consisted of six graduate students, and three renowned professors—a tipoff this wasn't a typical class. The initial lab lasted three hours.

The six of us sat in a semicircle within the one-story, cement-floored building. Black noiseless electronic recording devices covered one wall, and several enclosed cubicles with one-way windows were visible in the rear of the room. After brief introductions, the lead professor reminded us that the university's drop/add option remained available for three more days. It was clear the announcement was for our benefit. Only the professors and two senior graduate students who stood nearby knew what would soon take place.

Formalities and niceties concluded, we were led on a tour of several cottages all punctuated by a thick sweet smell as if the buildings' interiors had been deodorized to cover other smells. One cottage after another, we witnessed exceptional children the likes of which few people would ever see: children who watched a vinyl record spin endlessly on an antiquated player; children in wheel chairs who sat slumped and silent and by all appearances defeated; children who rocked ceaselessly staring at what only they knew; children who screamed and kicked at their cribs the moment we entered their cottage. None of the children spoke to us, not in words or functional gestures, raising the question whether they spoke at all. Few had the opportunity to move about. Most were confined to their undersized cribs, while others, removed from their cribs, were placed on the floor and secured by short tethers tied to a sturdy center post that supported the ceiling.

Two children wore boxing gloves to stop them from sucking on fingers that were raw. One boy walked the floor in a tight circle wearing a football helmet to prevent him from harming himself, we were told. (My earlier masters in clinical/counseling psychology failed to prepare me to fully grasp the phrase "harm himself." I'd be inalterably educated within the half hour.)

We returned to the lab in silence, the cottage experience numbing. We had been seated only moments when our attention was drawn to a young girl brought into the lab by a uniformed nurse who held firmly to the child's right wrist. The child was blonde, blue-eyed, skinny as a pencil, maybe six or seven years old, wearing a cute flowery dress. She walked on tiptoes as though she was dancing. She seemed very much alive and spirited. Her bright eyes suggested that she was happy, that she was in touch with her world and herself. Quite the contrast from the kids we had just seen. I offered her a smile, if not a tentative one. I had noticed that the nurse's expression was grim, the professors' as well.

A male graduate student who stood nearby moved forward and took hold of the child's right wrist, the exchange accomplished without a hitch—as if *any* hitch would have created a problem. With his secure hold on the child's wrist, the graduate student walked the youngster over to where we sat. Impishly, she brought her face close to each of us, peering into our eyes as though playing some enjoyable but unnamed game. She never said a word, never responded to our offered greetings. As she was now in front of me, feeling her breath, I was taken aback by the pronounced half-inch line of uninviting white tissue that divided her forehead. It ran from her hairline to the bridge of her nose, the chalky line noticeably pronounced against her tan skin. I stared at the line without premonition.

"She's been with us for three years, her parents unable to care for her," the major professor began, his tone somber. *Unable to care for her* pinned me to my seat. She looked so easy, so pleasantly child-like. Something was terribly wrong. "You've seen the scar tissue," the professor said, telling me what I should have known. "We've yet to discover how to prevent her from hurting herself. When she's alone, her arms must be restrained. That includes all through the night and most of everyday," he said, revealing his own frustrations. "Notice the darkened tissue at her chin. With her arms restrained, she would smack her chin against her shoulder, if permitted. She wears a neck collar during the night to prevent further damage."

The professor explained nothing else. He invited us to join him at a six-foot wide one-way window that was hidden behind a curtain. The nurse immediately moved to a door that opened to a secretive room visible through the window. The room was padded, and the spongy floor and walls covered with battleship gray canvas. The graduate student, his fingers firmly circling the child's wrist, walked the youngster into the room, leaving the door open.

The child entered willingly as if familiar with its confines, its procedures, and her task. She was light on her toes. A hint of a smile graced her lips, her eyes filled with their familiar brightness. Her left arm remained quiet at her sides; her narrow shoulders were relaxed. She might just as well have been on a picnic.

The graduate student moved the child to the center of the room. A rope with an attached dowel handle hung from its ceiling.

"We've tried teaching her to use her right hand for other purposes," the professor said, speaking of the hand the graduate student held. "By pulling the rope with her right hand a certain number of times—with no exhibited self-abuse, she earns treats she enjoys. The treatment has not been successful," he stated without passion. "Watch her right hand," he directed. Without pause, his voice weary, he said into a hidden microphone: "We're ready."

"We're ready," the graduate student replied, speaking for the child as well. He took a small step from the girl and released his grasp, leaving the child in her own space, a moment to enjoy her freedom.

The child's right arm and hand lay softly against her side, the deception brief. Without warning or change of facial expression, she coiled her right hand into a menacing fist, what she had been doing since she was three years old. As if controlled by an outside force, she brought her fist against the center of her forehead, against the thin line of scar tissue—the sound like a forceful hammer against a block of wood. The graduate student instantly grabbed the child's wrist preventing a second blow. That fast, with her wrist in the student's grasp, the child raised herself on her toes, her childlike dance returned as did her docile expression. With blood streaming from her forehead, her eyes, as before, sparkled.

Stunned into silence, we watched the nurse stem the blood while the child stood relaxed as if unfazed. If she were unfazed, she was the only person in the room so blessed. The nurse escorted her from the laboratory, returning her to her cottage and the jacket designed to restrain her thin arms against her meager chest.

The lead professor waited for her to leave before he took his seat. He wasted no time testing our convictions. "Is this how we wished to satisfy our professional lives? Are we prepared to commit ourselves to the task of helping these children improve their lives? Are we up to the challenge? Are we reliable? The children will test your skills," he warned. "They will test your patience," he promised. "They will test your endurance; they will test your commitment; they will count on you." He gave each of us a long, penetrating look. "Do you have any questions?"

When none of us spoke, he smoothed his voice and directed us, "Go home. Give what you've seen a chance to settle. Not everyone's suited to this work. You will earn my gratitude if you feel it wise to drop this lab. It's best you're not here unless you're entirely dedicated. There are other courses to take. Keep the image of this child in your mind as you consider your future. Your decision may affect her future as well."

Too upset to return to my apartment or the library, I chose to walk the grounds, the images of the child swirling in my mind. Without purpose beyond moving, I entered a three-story, administration building, its confines quiet as if most everyone had gone for the day. Off a hallway, I noticed an opened door and took a cautious step into a generously sun-filled room lined with large windows. I expected the room to be empty. I gazed left and froze. It seemed fate or chance needed to press me harder.

A bedded hydrocephalic child, perhaps five years of age, lay on his back in the room's farthest corner, the boy's immensely oversized head propped heavily on two pillows. He stared at me through large dark brown eyes. I felt my anger rise. As if I needed more evidence, the sight of the child shredded my previous delusion of fairness. I gazed at the child, helpless not to. I simply couldn't fathom what had happened that produced this end. To what purpose? I asked.

All these years later, I can still see the boy staring at me. I will not say to you that when his dynamic eyes and mine locked together, his did not implore. Despondent, I wished him goodbye and left impassioned and determined.

From the lab-course's first days, we were taught precision and patience and the realization that a child's smallest accomplishment could form the basis of prodigious growth.

We knew what we were expected to do: engineer solutions to help each child become more accomplished and confident every day. Further, we were to hold ourselves accountable, that is, improving a child's life was our responsibility. That realization left an indelible mark. We were to reject explanations that amounted to non-functional answers, where it was stated that a child's lack of progress was due to a faulty brain or a genetic error, inferred dynamics over which we had no control. We were to be self-regulating. If a child failed to progress, we were to change our tactics. Inadequacy was never attributed to the child, always to our strategies. That platform demanded and emboldened.

After weeks of intense lecture and demonstration, we were assigned children and goals to reach. In time, children who couldn't walk, walked, not necessarily three flights of steps, but enough to go independently beyond their cottage to enjoy what others took for granted. Many children who hadn't talked, talked, enough to visit a grocery store where they could manipulate their world by saying, "I want orange; I want milk." Children who would never read, read enough to find their name from the names of ten other cottage mates, enough to find their own labeled toothbrush, to look at picture books and discover with delight a recognizable word that transferred to a real object. Every child was a challenge, every child a puzzle to unravel, always the goal to help a child become stronger and more skilled.

It was impossible not to come away from the experience feeling empowered, with skills that provided a great sense of optimism, a confident perspective that most any difficulty a child presented, where time was not a yoke, was to some degree remediable. That attitude accomplished what was intended. It produced problem-solvers, not problem-namers.

As it was, I had become too comfortable, with theory and practice fitted within their proper location. I had left myself open for a confounding lesson with all the impact of a door slammed on a misplaced hand. Unexpectedly, life changed, and everything I had learned, everything I had prized professionally, came under challenge.

A SPECIAL SCHOOL, DENVER, CO

Shortly after earning my PhD from Arizona State, good fortune followed me to the University of Denver where I co-directed the graduate school psychology and educational psychology programs. It was the early 1970s, a time when fundamental and far-reaching changes were about to take place in both special education and general education, the results then felt no less than today. With my department head's approval, I accepted a psych-consultant position with a special school not far from the university's campus. To my great joy, it was as if the desert laboratory had moved with me to Colorado.

The facility was a cooperative school used by many surrounding school districts that sent us their most challenging children, thereby avoiding expensive duplication of services across districts. It made good economic and programmatic sense since the cooperative school assembled under the leadership of a forward-thinking principal several extraordinary speech and language pathologists, a remarkable physical therapist, and a company of outstanding special education teachers who were trained specifically for the complex children they served.

Our children were multiply handicapped, a fair term in those days— deaf and/or blind, self-injurious, speech and language involved, and orthopedically impaired. We had kids diagnosed with cerebral palsy, Down syndrome, and spina bifida, kids with infuriating, intractable seizures, children with inoperable brain tumors, and children with unusual genetic anomalies, some with devastating effects—e.g., Sanfilippo syndrome[1]—a metabolic disorder resulting in severe intellectual deficiencies and early death, the syndrome affecting several children from the same family, the youngsters and their parents always in my heart. We also served "idiopathic" kids, children whose symptoms had no known etiology—an *unnecessary* prerequisite to begin with in most instances. To my recollection,

there were no children described by their districts' special education directors as "autistic."

We did not choose which children attended the school. Districts made
those decisions. We had no problem satisfying a district's request to provide a unique program for any of their severely involved youngsters. We
had buckets of money thanks to a cryptic funding formula used to reim-
burse school districts for their low-incident handicapped children. We
could hire whatever staff we needed.

Our staff-to-student ratio was enviable. Most of our classes contained a
maximum of six to eight children. Several classes, for a brief time, had as
few as three children. Each class had at least one teacher and an aide. Our
classrooms were spacious and bright, and the children's large playground
was appointed with safe-play equipment. We had a multi-purpose gym
that during the day was never empty of kids, teachers, and therapists, especially the physical therapist.

The children, as diverse as they were, many with limited functional
communication skills, mixed well with each other. While they were taught
mostly in self-contained classrooms, they spent enjoyable times mixing
together throughout the day. No child was isolated for any length of time
from the others, and all the children interacted with our adult staff. More
so, the children were visited continuously by college students and younger
public school children, often both groups joining the special school's children in their classrooms, the visitors gladly put to work. With some license,
the special children at the Colorado school experienced a variation on
what special education knew as mainstreaming, a point that would soon
take on special significance as the following "FYI" will describe.

(FYI **A**: **Inclusion.** As the 70s ended, the federal concept of "least restrictive environment (LRE)"—"a gauge of the degree of opportunity a
person has for proximity to, and communication with, the ordinary flow
of persons in our society,"[2] gained momentum.

FYI **B**: **An error realized and rectified.** It was often customary to place,
for example, a non-verbal child into a self-contained classroom occupied by all non-verbal children, an administratively easy choice. It was
soon realized that grouping the similarly challenged children together
was a poor decision—if all the children were equally non-verbal, there'd
be no opportunity to model a speaking child thus, at the least, limiting
the possible acquisition of oral communication. Such glaring mistakes
no doubt fueled the fair and reasonable vision behind LRE.)

School districts, whether or not they approved the government's plan, adopted LRE. They had no choice if they wanted federal monies. Within several months, much to the disappointment of staff and parents alike, the self-contained, specialized Colorado school was closed, a decision made by the feeder districts' special education administrators who were acting within LRE's guidelines. The children once served at the cooperative school were dispersed to their individual home schools to be immersed within the population of general education pupils, the belief being that such inclusion would benefit the special children.

Shortly after the Colorado school's closure, at the behest of a parent of a former cooperative school pupil, I visited one of the schools where half a dozen transferred children were placed within the general education population.

As it turned out, the public school's officials had assigned the group of former Colorado special school children to their own small classroom space at the farthest end of a long hallway. Their lunch and outdoor recess were scheduled early when there'd be no contact with any other students but themselves, for their own safety, school officials claimed. By any measure, the move from the Colorado school to the public school was decidedly more restrictive. The children were kept from the general population, an example of LRE gone wrong. (The parents I spoke with were understandably incensed and gravely disappointed.)

Professionals working at the special school were not bound by any educational or psychological theory or current wave. Everyone's attention was directed toward each child's individual growth. Interventions were based on careful criterion assessment that relied almost exclusively on direct observation and in-class data collection rather than from standardized test numbers measured and provided by district school psychologists. Being told that a child had an 80 or 180 IQ, or a child was mildly retarded, provided us nothing that translated into effective strategies.

We had fashioned an ideal service delivery model, flexible enough to accommodate any unexpected request. I remember a call from one of the local special education directors, a strong advocate for all kids. "I have this child," he began. "She's 5, nonverbal, and has little interaction with anything outside herself. She suffers severe seizures that are frequent and uncontrolled despite medications. Nice parents. They're hurting. Put something together," he said, knowing it would be done within days.

The model was solutions oriented. We had virtually no encumbrances, no administrative edicts to follow—though we were required to submit formal categorical names/labels for districts to receive reimbursements.

The assigning of labels presented little problem since so few labels were used, most with some variation of "mental retardation." With the many cooperative parents who went out of their way to make our work easier and more successful, we found ourselves in an idyllic village with a singular purpose: to help the children become more successful across a wide breadth of skills and personal accomplishments.

From this scientist-practitioner's perspective, the Colorado special school, its children, their parents, and the staff, was a dream realized. As happens, however, dreams and some realities are without permanence. Priorities change, and programmatic scales shift their balance. Problems take on new perspectives, and professional adaptation becomes a necessary byword. As you'll see, the shift that occurred was nothing less than seismic.

THE NEW CHILDREN, CIRCA 1970s

In less than a decade, the ailment spread from virtual obscurity to something well beyond epidemic proportions. It has ... no universally accepted symptoms, and no discernible anatomical or biochemical characteristics which can be diagnosed in a clinic or laboratory. ... Before 1965, almost no one had heard of it, but by the beginning of the seventies it was commanding the attention of an armada of pediatricians, neurologists and educational psychologists, and by mid-decade, pedagogical theory, medical speculation, psychological need, drug company promotion and political expediency had been fused with an evangelical fervor to produce what is undoubtedly the most powerful movement in—and beyond—contemporary education.[3]

Dramatic changes were taking place within the public schools involving regular education children who weren't achieving as parents and teachers believed they should. Being told that some children struggled with reading and math did not surprise any of us at the Colorado school. We knew that the natural order of individual developmental differences, along with environmental variances, guaranteed such disparity. Discovering one bright morning that several of the surrounding districts had decided to send us their underachieving children astonished us.

The transferred children were an enigma. Bulging school reports preceded their arrival, reports that contained endless pages describing their academic *deficiencies*, replete with teacher accounts stating what a child *couldn't* do. We were confronted with new terms—at least new to us.

"Minimal brain dysfunction" and "diffuse organicity" were used freely as causal, underlying explanations for the children's math and reading deficiencies. The bulging folders and medical terminology seemed Shakespearean in proportion as if public school officials felt compelled to justify uprooting the pupils from their original schools and sending them to our self-contained facility.

Understand our confusion, if you will. After the staff and I read the public schools' narratives and vague references to brain injury, we'd glance toward our severely involved population as they struggled to say their names or balance on two frail legs or walk a wide hallway without suffering a seizure. The proposal that the newly arrived, socially engaging, highly verbal, obviously bright kids *had* brain damage said to be responsible for their poor classroom achievements was hard to accept. That the reports added the nebulous term "minimal" to the purported cerebral deficiency seemed preposterous, if not downright unethical.

The public school's decision to entrust us with the new children added to our consternation. Did they believe we possessed some tutorial magic that we had kept to ourselves? The implied message was that their districts' teachers lacked the competency to effect a change in a child's academic peculiarities. That, or the teachers felt intimidated by a child's proposed brain damage. This possibility struck us as strange, if not downright silly. The kids were just kids, after all.

Or was it something else? The cynic asked questions: Had regular education found a way to avoid individualizing instruction? Had regular education discovered that by sending the children to us it could reduce the number of students in its overcrowded classrooms? We had questions but few answers.

But we worked for the districts, and therefore we said nothing publicly other than "send us your kids and we'll provide for them." We hired teachers, we welcomed the children, and we did what we thought their home schools might have done:

1. Treat each child as an individual.
2. Identify academic strengths and where on a continuum those strengths broke down.
3. Assign children capable (flexible) teachers who allowed the children's progress to determine curriculum and strategies.

4. Maintain performance records examined weekly to assess the value of strategies.
5. Be self-regulating—change teaching strategies if the current one was unsuccessful.

In what seemed overnight, consensus was that most every capable child's classroom achievement struggles were a function of an organic error within the child, that virtually nothing else mattered. The groundswell in support of that newly founded belief was extraordinary, bandwagons across the country with standing room only. All that remained was to assign authoritative sounding names to the children's apparent abnormal physiological conditions and hope no one examined the biological scam, or the convenient educational nosology too closely.

- Under pressure, President Gerald Ford's federal government made promises it couldn't keep—and didn't fund.
- Congress, with help from the federal office of education, passed laws with grand notions (but without specifics enough to prevent confusion and multiple interpretations).
- A rejoicing regular education had a pipeline to move their troublesome children elsewhere.
- An egocentric special education turned its uncritical attention to its new population, a small number at first, a torrent to follow.
- Book publishers were awash in printed gold.
- Cottage industries sprung up everywhere: psychology with its testing, neurology with its diagnosing, pharmacology with its solutions.

There were doubters and dissenters, but the majority's zealous clamor drowned them out. Once the juggernaut's wheels began to turn, few in education looked back.

The overwhelmed, ill-prepared regular teachers had what they wanted.

The children without voices were moved like chess pieces.

Responsibility had shifted. A struggling child's biology was at fault. Nothing else. Talk about flimflam.

The dismayed Arizona ghosts looked on in silence.

NOTES

1. What is San Felipo Syndrome? (2017). *Team Sanfillipo*. Retrieved from http://teamsanfilippo.org/what-is-sanfilippo-syndrome.
2. Yell, M.L. (2010). Least restrictive environment, mainstreaming, and inclusion. Retrieved from http://www.education.com/reference/article/mainstreaming-inclusion/.
3. Schrag, P. & Divoky, D. (1975). *The myth of the hyperactive child and other means of child control*. New York: Dell Publishing Company.

CHAPTER 2

Disability Identification: The Naming Is Explaining Game

Several certainties are common to our respective fields. We're prone to declaring truths without adequate evidence. We talk more than we do. We find faults easier than we find solutions, and we have a penchant for placing individual kids within specified groups even though the children's remarkable (and predictable) diversity makes placement within these narrow clusters of little strategic importance. Despite this partiality that offers such minimal gains, we persist in our preoccupation to search out a categorical classification. Such discussions often dominate evaluations and interdisciplinary staff conferences as if everything depended on our collective agreement regarding which disorder's name to ascribe to a child. Some of us seem to believe that "could we but give the condition a name, the child would be saved."[1]

Practitioners who provide direct services to kids know the truth is more accurately characterized thusly. Stand ten youngsters in a line all labeled either "LD," "ADHD," "dyslexic," or "autism spectrum," and you'll have ten individual kids who require ten individualized behavioral and/or curriculum programs. Functionally, the categorical declarations serve federal government's tabulators and insurance companies, but few others. The downside is that the names we confidently agree upon are often interpreted to be real conditions that can cause real everyday school-related problems. The truth is much different.

In the late 1960s, arguing against our proclivities, a recognized authority in special education suggested with incisive simplicity that it would be

© The Author(s) 2017
J. Macht, *The Medicalization of America's Schools*,
DOI 10.1007/978-3-319-62974-2_2

best to define a child with a learning disability as "any learner who fails to benefit from an existing curriculum into which he has been placed."[2] If that prescription were followed, attaching the label to a child would be without controversy, and the wrangling and hours of dubious assessments dedicated to establishing the label's authenticity could be spent elsewhere. There's a secondary gain as well, one that could easily be considered the primary winner. The obvious intervention would be plain, incontrovertible, and applicable to virtually all the same labeled pupils: assess the child's academic entering skills, and modify the curriculum, both its content and its delivery. We could do exactly that when we first noticed a child struggling with his school work. Waiting for those struggles to worsen before we stepped in would be a gross error of the past. Supporting such an attitude, we were once similarly advised by a prominent psychologist: "We could forgo a categorical approach [and adopt] a fully dimensional, ... complaint-oriented approach [that] would better reflect the evidence."[3]

Today, given our recurrent debates about diagnostic classification and school-related disorders, it doesn't appear as if we're inclined to accept either reformist's suggestion toward the adoption of a non-categorical assistance delivery system that's based on needs, not names. In its place, we're left with what we have: special education's severely stressed eligibility system. That reality leads us to another discouraging certainty, specifically, our present funding limitations.

Considering our political priorities, and the way we educate our students, we're prevented from providing timely, effective services to all academically underachieving children. Since we likely agree that no truly needy youngster should be excluded for any reason from resource services, and since our restricted dollars need to be used as efficiently as possible, it's incumbent upon special education, for its own credibility, and school psychology, because of its diagnostic role, to possess a valid and reliable means to determine which children should be designated eligible for added assistance. A while back, the fear was expressed that if the two fields failed to discriminate accurately, a band of imposters would occupy most of special education's classroom desks, requiring that we turn away the rightful tenants.

A number of teachers will note readily that many, possibly most, of the "learning disabled" students enrolled in their programs do not satisfy either the 1977 USOE or the NJCLD definition. This is because, in many school districts, all students who are thought to be able to profit from tutoring or remedial education are arbitrarily called learning disabled. As a consequence of such definitional liberality, the learning disability programs have become glutted with underachieving students, culturally different students, and poorly taught students.[4]

We can't have that, can we?

Whether we possess such a valid and reliable means to make accurate eligibility decisions continues to be argued. While the *expectation* of such accuracy prevails, certainly among parents with needy children, eligibility decisions are compromised by factors that are beyond a diagnostician's ability to mitigate.

> Being declared eligible for special education services [has] less to do with the difficulties the child [is] experiencing with his or her school work, and more to do with the state and school district in which the youngster live[s].[5] When school districts have plenty of money to spend on educating students with disabilities, diagnostic personnel are encouraged to locate and identify as many students with handicaps as possible. When funds are limited, concerns grow about the large numbers of students being declared handicapped.[6]

The latter reality drew a warning from a 1990s note issued by a special education director:

> Special education is often the only available program for students needing some kind of classroom help. However, we must keep in mind that only students who are handicapped and in need of special education can be placed. Any student who does not meet the criteria is illegally placed and when we are monitored, we will have to payback any funds collected for an ineligible student. We can't afford to do this. Overall our numbers have increased by over 300 and we have added no more teachers. We cannot afford inappropriate placements, nor should we be labeling students as handicapped who are not.[7]

Budgetary matters, however, are the least problematic component that affects accurate identification of children with educational disabilities, one in particular that's especially daunting. Educational diagnosticians, when exploring core causes for a child's classroom difficulties, aren't measuring easily observed entities such as bacteria or white blood cells that lend themselves to numbers and precise communication. It's one thing to suggest that a defective heart has curtailed a child's athleticism. It's another to suggest that the same child's reading prowess is less than that of his classmates because of an educational disability known as "dyslexia." One offered explanation carries as a backup a series of lab markers. The other does not. One hypothesis can be verified and/or refuted. The other cannot. We've been forewarned.

> Drawing the line between normality and pathology is a contentious issue ...
> given the lack of objective "lab" markers. ...[8] Branding patterns of behavior
> as disordered will always have a cultural, value-laden component.[9]

It's easy to understand why our eligibility debates today are the same as they were over 50 years ago. The paradigm we use to make our judgments has changed little. We have the "medical model" to thank for our impasse. A closer look will reveal why.

EDUCATION'S MEDICAL MODEL

Medical causes for illnesses are based on what's known as "The Germ Theory," a fundamental tenet of the medical model. The theory states that microorganisms, which are too small to be seen without the aid of a microscope, can invade the body and cause certain diseases. Until the acceptance of the germ theory, many medical people believed that the diseases that plagued man were punishment for a person's evil behavior. When entire populations fell ill, the disease was often blamed on swamp vapors or foul odors from sewage. Even many educated individuals, such as the prominent seventeenth-century English physician William Harvey, believed that epidemics were caused by *miasmas*, poisonous vapors created by planetary movements affecting the Earth, or by disturbances within the Earth itself.[10]

Anton van Leeuwenhoek's and Robert Hooke's rudimentary microscopes dramatically changed medical thinking, providing science the means to observe, measure, validate, and refute what had never been seen, measured, or validated. With these advances, proof of organismic causes and contributors to disease and death were eventually established. Now visible directly, germs responsible for many of humankind's illnesses could be accurately and reliably diagnosed, providing the avenue for treatment and possible cure. The germ theory was established.

This effective model that answered so many troubling health-related questions could easily be adopted by other fields. Twentieth-century education was the ripest of the bunch.

Poorly performing schools have plagued the USA for years. Twice we've taken to dramatic and drastic measures to both identify and correct our educational deficiencies, one effort in progress today, what's known as "Common Core," and one that was mandated many years gone by. Memoire first, if you wouldn't mind, the implausible antecedent, a metal ball, 23 inches in diameter, weighing 184 pounds.

Not unlike today, the late 1950s and early 1960s were a time when many otherwise capable school children were underachieving in the classroom. The authorities then (as they are now) were determined to fix what they saw as a nation filled with student slackers. Today, our mandated all-encompassing change in school curriculum, namely, Common Core, has come about in part because of our own embarrassment derived from the world's perception that the USA is a third-rate educational country, resulting in, one might suppose, our academically impoverished children and their paltry standardized test scores:

> Reported in 2011. The U.S. was ranked 17th in an assessment of the education systems of 50 countries, behind several Scandinavian and Asian nations, which claimed the top spots. Finland and South Korea grabbed first and second places, ... Hong Kong, Japan and Singapore ranked third, fourth and fifth, respectively ... the U.K. ranked 6th, followed by the Netherlands, New Zealand and Switzerland ... Canada ranked 10th, followed by Ireland and Denmark. Australia, Poland, Germany and Belgium fared better than the U.S. on the top-20 list, which also included Hungary, Slovakia and Russia. The U.S. did better than Mexico, Brazil and Indonesia.[11] The World Economic Forum ranked the United States 52nd in the quality of mathematics and science education. That's ugly.
>
> (More current (2015), the U.S. ranks fourteenth (out of 40 countries) in "cognitive skills and educational attainment," 2nd (out of 14 countries) in ignorance of teen pregnancy, unemployment rates, and voting patterns, 24th out of 65 educational systems, 11th out of 50 countries in 4th grade math, and 6th (out of 49 countries) in 4th grade reading.)[12]

The ugly numbers demanded change. Conveniently, a historic event provided today's educational custodians their parochial solution, namely, tighten school curriculum.

OCTOBER 1957

Late in the afternoon of Friday, October 4, teletype machines around the globe screamed into motion. From Moscow came word that an artificial Earth satellite had been launched by the Soviet Union. The Soviet news agency Tass called the device Sputnik, a Russian nickname for "Artificial Fellow Traveler Around the Earth." The world's first man-made satellite and its instrumentation package ... circled the earth once every ninety-six minutes.[13,14]

National hysteria ran rampant. Predictions flew from all quarters that life, as we knew it, might soon cease. We little schoolkids did as we were told. We huddled shoulder to shoulder like chicks in a nest under spindly wooden tables in case the Russians, with their blinking, blanking satellite, dropped upon our elementary heads an atomic bomb.

Every politician who could speak spoke. Predictably, an inadequate US educational system was the designated punching bag.

> The Cold War stimulated the first example of comprehensive Federal education legislation, when in 1958 Congress passed the National Defense Education Act (NDEA) in response to the Soviet launch of *Sputnik*. To help ensure that highly trained individuals would be available to help America compete with the Soviet Union in scientific and technical fields, the NDEA included support for loans to college students, the improvement of science, mathematics, and foreign language instruction in elementary and secondary schools, graduate fellowships, foreign language and area studies, and vocational-technical training.[15]

Quite suddenly, the educational world we students had known for many years upended. With hardly any advance notice, as it happened, catching already jittery people ill-prepared, teachers mainly. Mostly, we young 'uns thought everything was fine, slow kids that we were, though we *were* smart enough to wonder what protection a meager wooden table would provide if the Russians were stupid enough to drop on our heads anything heavier than a paperclip.

By today's standards, of course, the Russian's high aerial act wouldn't earn a passing notice, not from those of us accustomed to watching intrepid astronauts play golf from the moon's natural bunkers, or catching glimpses from the Hubble Space Telescope as it views the fathoms of the universe. In 1957, the darn spherical object that nearly touched the hair on our feverish heads did scare the skiboddle out of us.

> Survival anxiety was all too real. Dr. Elmer Hutchisson, director of the American Institute of Physics, reacted to the events by suggesting that the nation's way of life might be "doomed to rapid extinction."[16]

Democratic Senator Henry Jackson of Washington described the feat as a "devastating blow" to the United States and called upon [then] President Eisenhower to proclaim "a week of shame and danger."[17]

An uneasy American public insisted on a whipping boy and a quick solution to what they saw as a catastrophic situation. *Sputnik* generated an intense educational crisis fueled by persistent criticism of our educational system. Reform of education to win the cold war became a temporary obsession in the media, in Washington, and throughout the country.

Sloan Wilson, author of the influential novel, "Man in the Gray Flannel Suit," and education editor of the New York Herald Tribune … asserted that [our] schools had "degenerated into a system of coddling and entertaining the mediocre."[18] Life magazine compared the schooling of two boys: one in Moscow and one in Chicago. It reported that in the Soviet Union, "The laggards are forced out [of school] by tough periodic examinations and shunted to less demanding trade schools and apprenticeships. … In contrast, American students lounge in classrooms that are 'relaxed and enlivened by banter,' and in which the 'intellectual application of [students] is moderate'."[19]

RISING STANDARDS[20]

We had become a paranoid populace, reminiscent of Peter Sellers's 1964 black comedy *Dr. Strangelove*. We had cement bomb shelters buried in our backyards. We were advised to stock these refuges with supplies sufficient to last—no one knew how long. In school, practice sessions were common where in the middle of geography class or the dreaded multiplication drills, an alarm rang and we'd be hurriedly led to the cafeteria or into the hallway to assume fetal positions under the earlier mentioned rickety table or pressed tight against a wall. Wrong as it was, I don't recall any of us taking the exercise too seriously. Twenty-five homeroom kids under tables, arms and legs interlocked, nervous giggles, making plans for after school. You get the picture.

The belief that *Sputnik* signified failings in America's educational system became widespread in late 1957. Americans seemed ready to accept the conclusion that the nation's scientific leadership, perhaps even survival, depended on changing its educational institutions. After *Sputnik*, achievement standards were increased, textbooks were rewritten, schoolwork became more formidable, expressly, "standards for reading achievement were raised and students were tested more rigorously."[21]

Predictably, students who hadn't performed well before the new standards didn't do an immediate 180-degree turn after the new standards were in place. Some students, prodded by parents, or by their own newly discovered need to excel, took to the more stringent curriculum without breaking a sweat. Others, however, routinely successful everyplace outside the classroom, knew they were lost academically. They faced requirements that were foreign and confusing, requirements for which they lacked basic understanding and thus the necessary prerequisite skills. The discrepancy between their classroom performance and the expectations others held for their achievements widened daily. In place of acknowledging that the newly raised standards for all might have left some students floundering, educational authorities, ever ready to protect their own derrières, opted for a more convenient, if not portentous, path, introducing into everyday conversation an ominous possibility. The medicalization of America's school child, what amounted to a catastrophic mistake, became a reality.

> Many children were unable to keep up with the new classroom requirements and the sharply elevated standards, but few blamed the rising of standards for the children's difficulties. Instead, students who scored low on reading achievement tests were personally blamed for their failure. ... If a child didn't satisfy the new demands ... the cause for the youngster's difficulties were "believed to be *organic*."[22] (Emphasis mine)

Education's affirmation that the roots of a child's school-based difficulties were organic fit the medical model so well that few people questioned its authenticity. With little objection, the concept of an organic educational germ that could explain a bright student's underachievement earned a spot alongside polio's virus, strep throat's bacteria, cerebral palsy's neurological base, and Down syndrome's genetic variation. Established now, poor reading, inadequate math skills, immature writing had its generalized categorical name, "learning disability," and its specific neurobiological cause, minimal brain dysfunction. Finally, an answer (Box 2.1).

Box 2.1 Medical model

Medical model

The **Medical** model assumes that a child's underachieving, inattentive behavior is caused by a neuro-biogenetic irregularity

---

This self-serving, expedited answer explained a child's underachievement well enough to satisfy the general populace, and a host of professionals who, astonishingly, were willing to overlook such insignificant details as follows:

- Education's proposed "germ" wasn't observable either directly or indirectly, thus making it just as likely to be fictional as fact.
- Education's applied "microscope" was a highly problematic set of psychometric (paper/pencil) exercises that were subject to the whims and judgment of the examiner, affected by the attitude of the individual being examined, and suffering its own content and construct validity issues, a significant departure from medicine's established diagnostic hardware and methodology that had successfully withstood multiple challenges to its authenticity.

Allow me to expound on that point a moment longer. Understand, please, that Pasteur's, Koch's, Leeuwenhoek's, and Robert Hooke's personal perspectives, agendas, and preferences did not affect the shape, size, or frequency count of their bacteria. The bacteria were either visible and measurable or they weren't visible and measurable, making accurate diagnostic predictions possible. In other words, Pasteur's diagnostic results and conclusions weren't influenced by an evaluator's bias or intentional data-manipulation, or by an examined subject's defiant attitude, often accompanied by the declaration, "I don't give a _ _ _ _ about your test."

Exacting measures and tight controls common to biological laboratories aren't part of today's classrooms or testing centers where chance and error affect most findings to some degree. Lumping together medicine's and education's use of the germ theory, as if they share empirical commonalities, comes with warnings. Notice the following conversation among diagnosticians who were charged with verifying the presence of a learning disability. How confident would we be if our family doctor played this loose with diagnosing what ailed us?

> *Psychologist 1:* [T]his is what puzzles me: Since there were no significant discrepancies, the [psychologist] determined that the ... scores must not be good scores ... so [he] chose to use the score on the cognitive test as an estimate of the [child's] OPTIMAL abilities. Using this score the examiner

could get a significant difference and say that a learning disability was present. ... My question is this: Is this a legitimate procedure? Is it appropriate to use a subtest score as the IQ score in computing a significant discrepancy [That's] like using a high score to say it was a more accurate reflection of a child's IQ when the other scores indicate otherwise?[23]

Psychologist 2: It is obviously a sham. The psychologist was going to find a learning disability [germ] no matter what instruments he/she administered or what the scores would be![24]

Psychologist 3: Yes. It's BS. No learning disability exists, in my opinion. ... The psychologist is looking for data to support his or her opinion, and disregarding what the actual data are showing that no learning disability exists! Highly unscientific, and perhaps bordering on unethical.[25]

Psychologist 4: Regarding IQs, ability/achievement discrepancy, LD, etc. I admit I've erred in using the term "throw outs" when discussing subtest scores. ... I started using the term "throwing out" instead of "partial out," which is not my intent or practice at all. We cannot "throw out" tests in the sense that we don't report them, i.e., pretend we never gave them.[26]

Psychologist 2: If we begin down the path of "partialling out" particular subtests scores ... what will keep unscrupulous (or merely stupid) practitioners from redefining ability ... in the service of their clients?[27]

Psychologist 4: I remain committed to the idea that when there is strong evidence that a cognitive weakness ... significantly affects ... an IQ score, it does indeed make sense to parcel it out. ... I believe there are times when it is necessary not to use a Full Scale score IQ.[28]

Psychologist 5: Perhaps the biggest issue regarding this topic is that of validity. What is it that we are measuring when we administer an individual intelligence test? If we are attempting to measure overall ability, then does not an individual's weaknesses enter into the picture? If the "goal" is to "find" a severe discrepancy so that the student may receive services, perhaps the ... model ... is at fault.[29]

Psychologist 3: Unfortunately, [these] procedures are not new to researchers who have investigated the use of LDs in practice. The procedure of shopping around until a discrepancy exists between some cognitive measure and ... achievement measures has been documented ... over the last 15 years. It has the same aura as setting monkeys loose with typewriters, finding coherent word or phrase and announcing the discovery of new intelligence.[30]

Summary: To be credible and trustworthy, the field of education must demonstrate that it can validly and reliably diagnose what it has chosen as its organic germ, what it uses to explain student underachievement and counterproductive behavior issues. Failure to do so, acting as if it possesses an accurate method when in fact it doesn't will inescapably generate serious doubts, complications, and faulty conclusions, the ramifications of the latter extensive. Which is precisely what has happened, distracting professionals and parents alike, leaving the waiting children to suffer the most. "Perhaps the model is at fault," the psychologist suggested. Perhaps it is. Let's find out.

NOTES

1. Smith, R.M. & Neisworth, J.T. (1975). *The exceptional child: A functional approach.* New York: McGraw-Hill.
2. Barsch, R.H. (1968). Perspectives on learning disabilities: The vectors of a new convergence. *Journal of Learning Disabilities, 1,* 7–23.
3. See Spitzer, Robert L., M.D., Williams, Janet B.W., D.S.W., First, Michael B., M.D., Gibbon, Miriam, M.S.W., Biometric Research; Maser, J.D. & Akiskal, H.S. et al. (2002) Spectrum concepts in major mental disorders *Psychiatric Clinics of North America,* Vol. 25, Special issue 4; Krueger, R.F.; Watson, D.; Barlow, D.H. et al. (2005). "Introduction to the Special Section: Toward a Dimensionally Based Taxonomy of Psychopathology". *Journal of Abnormal Psychology* 114 (4): 491–493. doi:10.1037/0021-843X.114.4.491. PMC 2242426. PMID 16351372; Bentall, R. (2006). "Madness explained: Why we must reject the Kraepelinian paradigm and replace it with a 'complaint-orientated' approach to understanding mental illness." *Medical Hypotheses* 66 (2): 220–233. doi:10.1016/j.mehy. 2005.09.026. PMID 16300903.
4. Myers, P.I. & Hammill, D.D. (1990). *Learning disabilities: Basic concepts, assessment practices, and instructional strategies* (3rd ed.) (p. 13). Austin, TX: PRO-ED.
5. Reynolds, C.R. (1990). Conceptual and technical problems in learning disability diagnosis. In C.R. Reynolds & R.W. Kamphaus (Eds.), *Handbook of psychological and educational assessment of children: Intelligence and achievement* (p. 574). New York: Guilford.
6. Ysseldyke, J.E., Algozzine, B., & Thurlow, M.L. (1992). *Critical issues in special education* (p. 350). Boston: Houghton Mifflin Company.
7. Personal Communication: Memo from Executive Director of Special Education and Pupil Services to School Psychologists (1992), Tucson, AZ.
8. Hinshaw, S.P. & Scheffler, R.M. (2014). *The ADHD explosion: Myths, medication, money, and today's push for performance* (p. 18). New York: Oxford Press.
9. Wakefield, J.C. (1992). The concept of mental disorder. On the boundary between biological facts and social values. *American Psychologist, 47,* (3), 373–388.
10. Kusinitz, M. (2017). Germ theory. *Net Industries.* Retrieved from http://science.jrank.org/pages/3035/Germ-Theory.html.

11. Gayathri, A. (2012). US 17th in global education ranking; Finland, South Korea claim top spots. *International Business Times*. Retrieved from http://www.ibtimes.com/us-17th-global-education-ranking-finland-south-korea-claim-top-spots-901538.
12. Rice, M. (2014). Ranking America: a site for information about the U.S. Retrieved from https://rankingamerica.wordpress.com/category/education/.
13. Clowse, B.B. (1981). *Brainpower for the cold war: The sputnik crisis and national defense education act of 1958* (p. 28). Westport, CT: Greenwood Press.
14. Garber, S. (2007, October 10). Sputnik and the dawn of the space age. *NASA History Web*. Retrieved from https://history.nasa.gov/sputnik. See also: https://en.wikipedia.org/wiki/Sputnik_1.
15. The federal role in education. (2017). *Department of education*. Retrieved from http://www2.ed.gov/about/overview/fed/role.html.
16. Clowse, B.B. (p. 21). (See also: A birthday flexing of red biceps. (1957, November 18.) *Life*, p. 35, and Building brainpower. (1957, November 4). *Newsweek*, p. 96).
17. Jackson, H. (1957, October 6). Blow to U.S. seen. *New York Times*. Retrieved from http://www.nytimes.com/1957/10/06/archives/blow-to-us-seen-jackson-says-soviet-satellite-hurts-nations.html.
18. Clowse, B.B. (1981). p. 106. See also Wilson, S. (1958, March 24). It's time to close the carnival. *Life*, 37.
19. Sleeter, C.E. (1986). Learning disabilities: The social construction of a special education category. *Exceptional Children*, 53, 46–64.
20. Macht, J. (1998). *Special education's failed system*. Westport, CT: Bergin & Garvey.
21. Sleeter, C.E. (1986), p. 46.
22. Sleeter, C.E. (1986), pp. 46–64.
23. 96-07-09 PSYCHOEDUCATIONAL_ASSESS.
24. Tue, July 9, 1996-0400 PSYCHOEDUCATIONAL_ASSESS.
25. Tue, July 9, 1996-0600 PSYCHOEDUCATIONAL_ASSESS.
26. Fri, November 17, 1995-0500 ASSESS-P.
27. Mon, November 9, 1995 ASSESS-P.
28. Fri, November 17, 1995 ASSESS-P.
29. Wed, November 15, 1995-0700 ASSESS-P.
30. Tue, July 9, 1996 PSYCHOEDUCATIONAL_ASSESS.

CHAPTER 3

Learning Disabilities

CURRICULUM *RIGOR MORTIS*

If a child struggles with schoolwork, if he or she underachieves in the classroom, if a teacher (or parent) hopes to arrange resource (special education) assistance, the youngster will need to be designated eligible for those services.

Most often, the eligibility process is an extended, twisting maze where the fiscal goal of the exercise is to deny the child services, money being the obvious malefactor. Because of finances, some states cap the number of children they are willing to serve, which, in effect, prevents children who need services from receiving them. A Texas mother recently told a federal hearing committee, "Educators called my daughter cute and sweet but ignored her learning needs. My child is seven, and she can't identify the word 'the,' and that's wrong." A special education teacher speaking at the same committee hearing shared, "Oftentimes when it was very, very obvious that a child needed services, I would go through the steps required and they [the school eligibility committee] would say, well, 'Let's wait six weeks, eight weeks and see how they do.' ... So by the time [the children] do get tested, they've lost all that time for support." Yet another pleaded, "The schools are not meeting [the children's] needs. You need to change that. You really do. This just cannot keep going on."[1]

© The Author(s) 2017
J. Macht, *The Medicalization of America's Schools*,
DOI 10.1007/978-3-319-62974-2_3

Why did the Texas mom and the special education teachers face such resistance? The answer's simple, though not satisfying. Schools (and related federal government agencies) are looking for ways to reduce special education's rolls. Why the pressing need to make it harder for kids to get services? Remember what the special education director said in the previous chapter? "Special education is often the only available program for students needing some kind of classroom help." Then she added, "Any student who does not meet [eligibility] criteria is illegally placed and when we are monitored, we will have to payback any funds collected for an ineligible student. We can't afford to do this."

"Q": Why is special education the only hand at the player's table? There are other seats available, one clearly reserved for regular education. "A": The answer might surprise you. Since the 1970s, regular education has been granted tacit permission to excuse its perennially underperforming classroom from any culpability when it comes to a child's weak scholastic achievement. That's sort of like excusing the US Congress for writing an indecipherable tax code that appears to have intentionally been written in Greek. Any other business (or institution) with the same record would have folded under its own futility.

Quickly, we shouldn't fault regular education entirely for its lack of effort to either monitor or improve its own unwieldy system. After all, the field is simply taking full advantage of the gift that was bestowed. Make no mistake: we brought much of the current educational morass on ourselves when we reasoned that a youngster's inability to succeed with his curriculum was due to his "organic" problem. That choice pleased many a vanquished teacher, and made lots of neurologists rich and happy. The expedient decision has been haunting us for years.

A small, rural school close to my office has seventy-six third graders, divided among three classes. Twenty-four of the third-grade children have been referred and found eligible for special education services, either for learning disabilities or speech and language difficulties, the latter used in place of learning disabilities to obtain special education assistance with reading and writing assignments.

During the second week of the school year, one of the third grade teachers announced she intended to refer ten additional students from her class for special education evaluation. The teacher reported the children were not prepared for their third grade spelling assignments; the teacher stated the children should be taught in a smaller group where they could receive individual assistance. (The total cost for evaluation and assessment for the new ten referrals will approach $15,000 to $18,000.)

Chances are that only five or six of the teacher's ten will meet special education criteria, bringing the total of special education third graders to twenty-nine out of the original seventy-six. If only five children are found eligible for special education, the third grade will have 38% of its students enrolled in special education[2] —The late Reed Martin, author, lawyer, special education advocate.

The above is not an exaggeration. In the late 1980s, I was summoned by a Denver school principal to discuss a youngster who was creating problems for himself, his teacher, and his fellow students. During the conversation, the suddenly maddened administrator took an abrupt detour. With smoke rising from her scalp, she explained that one of her kindergarten teachers had just referred half her class of 20-some children for special education evaluation because of their poor writing skills. The regular education teacher was thoroughly convinced the children were disabled. She didn't know what it was, only that *it* was. I chose not to ask the principal, "It was what?" She and I looked at each other in utter dismay. Half of her mostly five year olds referred because of immature writing? I was disheartened less by the teacher's incredible conclusion than how she arrived at it. History will provide some insight.

Until protective federal laws were passed in 1975, America's recalcitrant educational system instructed only one out of five children with identified disabilities (e.g., deaf/blind, cerebral palsy [CP], retardation). At the end of World War II, our public school system had settled comfortably atop its own empire, holding tight-fisted the power to decide who could and who couldn't enter its revered classrooms. Children judged atypical or less than average were denied entrance, their parents without recourse or reasonable alternatives.

Until the mid-1970s, laws in most states allowed school districts to refuse to enroll any student they considered "uneducable," a term generally defined by local school administrators.[3]

In 1970, a task force studying students from the Boston school area "found over ten thousand students excluded from public school classrooms because they didn't match school standards for the normal student."[4] Later in the decade, it was estimated that well over a million school-age children were refused access to public schools and another 3.5 million children received little to no effective instruction simply because "they were different in some way."[5,6] One state supreme court justified excluding a young boy with cerebral palsy because he "produce[d] a depressing and nauseating effect upon the teachers and school children."[7] Many states had laws that explicitly excluded children with certain types of disabilities, including children who were labeled "emotionally disturbed" or "mentally retarded."[8] Markedly different children mostly found themselves isolated in institutions, secluded in basements of churches, or left to remain in their homes rather than seated inside public schools with qualified teachers at the tiller. The public schools' endearing message: Those kids and their parents would have to find their own educational facilities.

In the 70s, at my younger children's elementary school, I recall how school officials debated enrolling a wheelchair-bound child, the youngster eight or nine years of age, a victim of a recent horrendous automobile accident where he was propelled through the windshield of his mother's car when a drunk driver ran a red light. How would the children respond to such a sad sight? That was the question raised by a troubled administration. Were they doing the other children a disservice by exposing them to this different child? Would the children be so taken aback that they'd ignore the youngster altogether? Not surprisingly, the school children instantly welcomed the boy as one of their own, several hoping to catch a ride in his big-wheel chariot.

Some of those different kids *did* attend public schools in the 1960s and 1970s. They had the good fortune to carry on their person a favored passport that allowed unchallenged passage beyond the school building's front door. Their good fortune? They didn't flail insubordinate arms, or sit with dangling, lifeless legs, or gaze with moon faces, half-closed eyes, and drooling mouths. In other words, they appeared like all the other pleasant-looking children.

Most of the fortunate children were cordial and cooperative, and their days in the school room passed with little additional teacher attention needed or offered. That is until they faced the instructor's preplanned curriculum and accompanying exams with questions and exercises that were the same for all the children. It was then that those children separated themselves from the others by their lack of success with their studies. It was then that their presence was noticed, as was the burden their differences created for the general educational system whose less compassionate teachers treated childhood diversity as if it were an infectious disease.

Public school administrators largely ignored parental pleas for help with the children who wrestled with their basic studies despite the parents' earnest testimonies that their children were supremely capable with so much in their lives. Only in school did they falter, the parents explained. "That means something, doesn't it?" they asked. It was a question school officials were not yet ready to hear, much less consider.

When the parents tried convincing family, friends, or school administrators that their children must be suffering from a "mysterious neurological handicap, a chemical imbalance, or a quirky syndrome,"[9] they were met with unsympathetic ears and suspicious stares. Their related stories were heartrending, true confessions that told of a concerned mother defending her child against the bureaucratic intolerance of a school system:

> Overriding all else was the feeling of helplessness brought on by indifferent authorities who were quick to declare that the children were either lazy or retarded—or the product of ignorant or disturbed parents.

Know that those worried 1960s parents weren't slackers, too busy celebrating their own pampered lives to know and appreciate the challenges their children were experiencing in school. To the contrary, they were by and large middle-class, suburban, and college-educated, good parents, good citizens, veterans of the League of Women Voters or the Parent Teacher Association (PTA) or the American Association of University Women (AAUW). And they shared with one another similar horror stories, stories of their misunderstood children, of teachers who threw up their hands in despair, of pediatricians who had no referrals or suggestions, of psychologists who misconstrued and misdiagnosed.[10] Parents lamented, "You felt like you were all alone … [that] no one could help." Most demoralizing was that "educators made you feel like your child was a freak," and "almost every [parent] was told their children's school problems were emotionally caused, that the children's learning difficulties were the mother's fault." One mom conceded, "As someone who thought she was doing a good job as a mother and had been a good elementary teacher, it was a real trauma to be told I had given my child an emotional block to learning. ... Even though it wasn't true ... I had all this guilt. That was the worst part," investigative reporters Peter Schrag and Diane Divoky recounted. Frustrated, even angered, at the reception they and their children received from the schools, the parents in their darkest moments held tightly to their convictions that something unknown or undetected was interfering with the children's scholastic efforts.

It was a desperate time for the parents. They were determined to finally free themselves from professional charges that their children's learning problems were caused by what was happening at home. Intuitively, they knew otherwise. But they faced deaf ears and minds as impenetrable as marble. They needed help. They needed an answer with clout. They needed a standard-bearer, someone who would provide an explanation for their children's struggles, a documented answer from an authority, some attestation they could carry to school officials and state audaciously, "Listen up you bleeping bleep bleep. Here's *why* my kid's having such a hard time learning. It's not his fault. It's not my fault. Stick that...on your bulletin board." The answer would be theirs sooner than then they thought possible.

CHICAGO, 1963

On April 6, 1963, a resourceful group of flustered parents convened a conference in Chicago entitled "Exploration into the Problems of the Perceptually Handicapped Child." Participating professionals came from various disciplines, many with diverse and extensive clinical experience with capable children who struggled with their classwork. Yet, despite their academic credentials, they, too, lacked a cohesive answer that could explain why bright children would have problems reading, completing math assignments, or following at times what seemed to be simple directions. Their questions mirrored those of the children's parents, particularly one that asked: How could a child be so proficient at one task and have such difficulty with another?

One of the conference's speakers was Professor Samuel Kirk, a psychologist and noted researcher and educator. One might fairly speculate that he didn't realize the far-reaching history he was to make that day, the extent of which reverberates today.[11] In moments, he would with the fewest of words dramatically influence special education and much of school psychology's present and future. After sharing some of his work with the audience, he made a kindly offer. To those gathered, Sam Kirk said something to the effect of "I've coined the term 'learning disabilities,' a term a colleague and I have mentioned in various papers. I've used it to *describe* a group of children. If it will be of any help, you're welcome to use it."[12,13] (Emphasis mine.)

It didn't take long for Dr. Kirk's words to brew to their full flavor. Those in the audience heard what they needed to hear, what they wanted to hear. The parents heard Sam Kirk say the word "disabilities." The parents thought they heard the word "condition." They thought they heard Sam Kirk say, "their children had a condition," a malady no less in kind than asthma or chicken pox. The parents came to the conference seeking an explanation for their children's school failings. Professor Kirk's "learning disabilities," though a created term he had mentioned in a few papers, provided an immediate benefit best voiced by an elated mom when, from the heart, she confessed, "Once we knew we had this special [learning disabilities, LD] problem, all the guilt vanished."[14]

Before the Chicago conference ended, the participants decided by consensus that "learning disabilities" would represent a new disability category, the parents convinced the term epitomized the uniqueness that best described their own children, one that importantly distinguished their youngsters from others who were said to be mildly mentally retarded and/ or emotionally disturbed. By the time Sam Kirk left the podium, learning disabilities, gaining power by the moment, had established its own footing and its own space.

Influenced by pressure from parents and professionals, the federal government passed legislation for the benefit of the children said to be learning disabled.[15] Five years after Sam Kirk's inauguration, the feds designated "specific learning disability" an approved disability category (US Office of Education, 1968) (The committed grammatical error went mostly unrecognized. Please see below.) Special education, by its own choice, would never be the same. With language embedded in Sam Kirk's "learning disabilities," parents around the USA who shared similar concerns regarding their children's schooling found each other without effort. By the mid-70s, they formed hundreds of local and state organizations enrolling more than 45,000 members, and adding up to 5000 new members a year. They talked to medical and educational communities, drumming up support for what they were certain was the solution to their problems, understandably believing that...

...[i]f, could they but give the condition a name, the child would be saved.[16]

Medical people saw what was happening. A few understood the new term's financial possibilities. Several physicians aligned themselves with the advancing advocacy groups lending more credibility to the movement. Talk was that large numbers of children across the USA fit within the developing LD rubric. In the 1970s, Eric Denhoff, a pediatric neurologist and paid LD spokesman, suggested that "at least ten percent of children from middle-class homes [were] learning disabled. With children from lower socioeconomic families," Denhoff suggested, "the percentages [were] much higher."[17] Excitement permeated the physician's prediction. After one special education staffing, I witnessed parents hugging the attending staff, thanking them for designating their child disabled. It seemed surreal. In my experience, "disabled" and "joyful appreciation" rarely occupied the same galaxy.

The LD movement grew and hopes abounded. Sam Kirk's term acquired its own healing properties. It soothed parental fears, and it mitigated parental doubts. Foremost in the parents' minds, it ended the unbearable silence that came with their not knowing *why* their children struggled so. They had their categorical name; they had their sought after explanation.

(FYI: No one thought to tell the parents otherwise, to suggest that the yearned for answer as they envisioned it was hampered by serious impediments. Had someone done so, had the parents been cautioned that they might have misinterpreted what Dr. Kirk said, the parents would not have heard the warning. They had waited so long for what they now had that their interpretation, despite its failings, mattered more than what was accurate. Fifty years later, the same attitude often holds true, the resulting consequences soon to become evident.)

NUMBERS

Early on, the numbers of children said to be learning disabled were relatively few, hardly enough to evoke much notice. In 1975, when the Education for All Handicapped Children Act (Public Law 94-142 [94th congress,] 142nd bill) was signed into law by the then president, Gerald Ford, federal costs required to assist the children newly designated as exceptional was accepted as necessary and politically correct. The federal government's spokesperson let it be known that "[c]ost was not an issue. The social value of ideals outweighed funding considerations."[18] That philanthropic attitude was about to change abruptly. A disability that had not officially existed before 1963 soon became a major presence.

(FYI: To know how often an event occurs, the one who keeps count must know what s/he's counting? You can, for example, visit zoos and count the number of aardvarks basking in the sun. The creature's been photographed, which helps if you've never seen an aardvark. That special education had yet to develop a means to confirm or deny the presence of the new disability, much less take its picture, didn't dissuade the federal government from compiling its figures.)

The following federal government's compiled LD numbers are only guesstimates. The actual numbers are unknown and will always remain so. The reasons in part being that

[t]he federal government ... failed to provide the professional special education community a satisfactory method to either confirm or deny the presence of the new disability.[19] Outspoken others, were more pointed. Writing in the 1978 Journal of Learning Disabilities, they doubted that a "technically sound solution to the problem of LD identification even existed."[20]

In 1968, 120,000 children were *designated* learning disabled. In 1977, the number increased to 796,000. In 2003, the number neared 3 million.[21]

(**FYI A**: Currently, it is estimated that there are 2.4 million American public school students (approximately 5% of the total public school enrollment) officially identified as learning disabled. This reduction in frequency counts might be better understood when considering the increased numbers of students who have qualified for special education assistance under the rubric of speech and language disorders and/or autism. The phenomenon is known as "diagnostic substitution" where children, no longer found eligible to receive special education services under other diagnostic categories—specifically speech impairment and learning disabilities—are now being served under the autism spectrum disorder [ASD] category.[22] **FYI B**: Supporting the earlier "substitution" observation, rates of reported autism increased by more than 20-fold when the diagnosis of ASD became a prerequisite for extra school services.[23,24] Schools began to include autism as a special education classification in 1992.[25] Returning to the 2015 government study, its author, Micelle Diament, writing for *Disability Scoop*, reported: "In some cases, parents admitted that clinicians gave their child an autism diagnosis simply because that label would make [school] services more readily available." **FYI C**: Those of us who believe that all children should have access to resource services have no problem with the naked duplicity.)

When Sam Kirk's term first began to appear in schools' eligibility hearings, the issue of denying or confirming the presence of a learning disability did not gain much attention from professionals in special education, or from the "bean counters" in Washington. Again, the numbers of children so designated were few. Still, those children said to be learning disabled did receive services, and those services did cost federal dollars.

In the late 1970s, when identified LD kids exceeded 500,000, Congress realized it had no handle on the numbers of children who might qualify for special education assistance. Authoritative testimony presented during legislative hearings estimated that as many as 40% of the present school-age population could be classified as learning disabled depending upon which definition was adopted. A decade later, authorities suggested that "by using the various measurement models employed among the states, 'an astute diagnostician can qualify between 50% and 80% of a random sample of the population as having a learning disability that requires special education services'."[26] Since every eligible child would receive some amount of funding, the dollar costs were potentially staggering,[27] which is an accurate assessment. In 1975, federal special education costs were a mere $250 million dollars. In fiscal year 2014, federal costs were $12.50 billion dollars, with $11.45 billion of that going to state grants. LD received the major share of the budget at 42% of the funds, speech and language impairments received 25%, and autism spectrum received 9%— the three accounting for 76% of the federal funds.[28] The real costs, however, were (and are) unknown. The current federal contribution of $12 billion represents a small portion of the total cost of today's special education. In perspective, during the 1999–2000 school year, the feds' share of funding was only 9% of the total cost. The states covered 45% and the local districts covered 46%. Collectively, in the school year 1999–2000, total regular and special education spending on students with disabilities was estimated at $77.3 billion dollars.[29] Today's costs most certainly are higher. The practical effects of these astonishing costs extended into school programs outside the boundaries of special education. In the years following the steady rise of students found eligible for additional services, school systems struggled to find a solution to the perplexing dilemma it faced every day. In the 1990s, costs became acute.

> While special education spending continues to grow, [federal] funding has not kept up, forcing school administrators to 'encroach' upon general education revenues to pay the costs of special education. Over a quarter of all special education program expenditures in California, on average, are paid from a school district's general fund. ... In 1991–92, the special education program in Los Angeles incurred a deficit of $154 million—a deficit recovered through nonmandated encroachment into the school district's general fund.[30]

In the summer of 2010, the New Jersey's *Star-Ledger* ran a hard-hitting piece about the condition of education finance in the Garden State. It bemoaned a dismal school-system budget in which teachers had been laid off, extracurricular activities scrapped, and free transportation curtailed. But one budgetary category had been spared: special education. Larrie Reynolds, superintendent in the Mount Olive School District where special education spending rose by 17% this year, said:

> This is an area that is completely out of control and in desperate need of reform. Everything else has a finite limit. Special education—in this state, at least—is similar to the universe. It has no end. It is the untold story of what every school district is dealing with.[31]

The following point did not go unnoticed:

> Schools, districts, and states ... face challenges in identifying special education students, both to determine who requires additional services and to calculate the costs of their education. In contrast to the identification of other at-risk children, such as those in poverty, special education determinations require expertise, judgment, and a level of subjectivity. Because federal subsidies for special education total $11.5 billion per year and schools themselves are at the center of the identification process, financial incentives can encourage schools to identify students as requiring special education who may not, in fact, need those services.[32]

From a monetary point of view, costs to serve the numbers eventually caught the eye of the federal government as well as the states' accountants, the latter who slept soundly only when their budgets balanced. By the mid-1980s, it was estimated that some 1000 people per day were being told they were learning disabled.[33] Ten thousand might be closer to the truth given the term's casual and curious use to explain a wave of everyday concerns:

"LD [has been] used to explain all sorts of deviant cognitive, academic, and social activities not originally intended, including not being able to\find one's car in a shopping mall's parking lot." The late William M. Cruickshank, honored professor, author, and special education advocate, related, "Parents in their concept of learning disability have talked to me about nail biting, poor eating habits, failure of the child to keep his room neat, unwillingness to take a bath, failure to brush teeth. Teachers have questioned me about disrespectful children, children who will not listen to the adult, children who are sexually precocious, children who are aggressive—all in the belief that these are learning disability children. One parent asked me if the fact that his college-student son wore long hair and he 'suspected' lived with a girl outside his dormitory was the result of a learning disability."[34]

LD IDENTIFICATION

By their inaction, [the feds] left the ground-breaking 1975 Education for All Handicapped Children Act (Public Law 94-142) hanging with its inherently vague and imprecise LD definition that was difficult to put into actual practice.[35]

[T]he entire concept of learning disabilities is dated and flawed. With enough testing, close to half the population can be classified LD; with money attached to the classification there is a lot of impetus to put any kid that needs more help into LD programs, particularly in resource-strapped schools. The model comes out of 1950s and 60s thinking ... and is so outdated as to be embarrassing.[36]

There is no clear and widely accepted definition of learning disabilities. Because of the multidisciplinary nature of the field, there is ongoing debate on the issue of definition, and currently at least twelve definitions appear in the professional literature.[37]

A growing number of professionals within special education, including school psychologists upon whom often fell the responsibility to determine LD eligibility, were frustrated by the lack of eligibility structure and direction. Parents particularly were unhappy. In the absence of a precise means to determine a learning disability, these guardians were often the recipients of unfavorable eligibility decisions that seemed more random than qualified. Increasingly, disgruntled parents whose children had been rejected by special education brought divisive and expensive litigation against schools. School districts who may have wanted to do right by the kids were often reduced to ping pong balls batted around by savvy lawyers and a federal doctrine that had no bones, much less teeth. Even the winners lost—as did many of the children who were pawns in what often dissolved into an acrimonious contest. In effect, the special education feds in Washington sent the local school's diagnostic team stumbling into the LD-eligibility mine shaft without so much as a candle, much less a lantern or a canary. It was one thing to categorize and designate a child as learning disabled. It was another to know if the designation was accurate. It was not an easy time for a generous field that prided itself on providing a safety net for virtually all children regular education routinely abandoned. Nevertheless, frugal eyes kept watch as special education searched out an unerring diagnostic procedure for its coveted "learning disabilities."

> With great reluctance by many, special education adopted a categorical discrepancy definition. This definition has been soundly criticized on almost every conceivable ground *except* undue exclusion of children.[38]

As it happened, the parents who attended the 1963 Chicago convention unknowingly offered special education the foundation upon which to build its diagnostic methodology. The parents had witnessed their own children's poor achievement, and they were certain their offspring were more than capable of doing better. There within that realization was the telltale incongruity special education would use to track down an LD, summed up by a simple axiom:

- Intelligent children should do well in school.
- Failure of intelligent children to do well in school must mean the children suffer from a disability.

It made sense, as do most self-evident truisms when seen at first blush. With a second more objective take, the axiom might have warranted a significant modification.

Special education thought to substantiate the presence or absence of an LD with two numerical measures: the level of a child's classroom achievements and the measure of that child's innate ability or intellectual potential.

- The LD benchmark would be as follows:
  A child would be designated LD if he or she possessed high *innate* ability (as defined by an intelligence quotient [IQ] score), while failing to exhibit classroom achievement at a level that the IQ (or the parents or teachers) predicted.
- The non-LD benchmark would be as follows:
  A child with low *innate* ability (as defined by an IQ score), regardless of achievement level attained, would fall within the non-LD category.

The eventual diagnostic model adopted by special education was known as the "IQ–Achievement Discrepancy Model,"[39] where the term *discrepancy* represented an unexpected observation regarding a child's school performance given his or her ability level. Basically, special education (and parents) assumed that children with high innate intelligence would achieve well in school. A child with high intelligence who did not achieve well in school would, *ipso facto*, exhibit a discrepancy. Therein lies the basis of the IQ–Achievement *discrepancy* model.

Special educator Barbara Bateman had witnessed bright children struggling mightily with their school work—precisely what the 1963 parents had observed with their own children. In 1965, Dr. Bateman introduced her IQ–Achievement discrepancy that boasted the two key components special education needed: "estimated intellectual potential and actual level of classroom performance."[40] Some ten years after Bateman's model was introduced, the federal division of special education made the IQ–Achievement discrepancy model official. It stipulated that

[a]n interdisciplinary team may determine that a child has a specific learning disability if: (1) The child does not achieve *commensurate* with his or her age, [or exhibits] a discrepancy between his or her achievement and intellectual

ability (USOE, 1977, p. 65083). Thus, the IQ-Achievement discrepancy was established as the primary criterion for LD identification. Over time, it became almost the exclusive variable used for LD eligibility determination.[41] (Emphasis mine)

Special education and school psychology made the assessment process simple. Almost universally, they used the same two standardized tests across the country: one that claimed to assess a child's classroom achievement (the Woodcock–Johnson Achievement Test) and one that claimed to measure innate intelligence (the Wechsler Intelligence Test for Children [WISC]).

(**FYI**: "Standardized" means all examined children receive the same instruments administered in the same manner regardless of their background, culture, language skills, the skills of their teachers, their classroom curriculum, their parental support, or their environmental history. None of those elements should matter much if we were assessing something that's proven to be *innate*, part of a child's biological makeup, an attribute *not* strengthened or weakened by environmental influences. *Innate* intelligence should qualify as such an attribute. On the other hand, these same elements, background, culture, language skills, and the like, would certainly matter if we were assessing a characteristic that is alterable by daily experiences, school skills, for example, such as vocabulary, number sense, puzzle solutions, the same stuff a youngster can find on the back of a cereal box and anywhere else with a smart phone.)

INNATE INTELLIGENCE

Though we'll only discuss the intelligence factor, recognize that if the instruments special education and school psychology use to measure either a child's classroom achievement or the youngster's intelligence have prompted serious validity concerns, then the essential discrepancy component used in special education's discrepancy model is called into question, if not flat-out compromised. Specifically, we're concerned with the possible lack of what psychologists call "construct"[42] and/or "content validity"[43]—the latter particularly important since it speaks to what teachers presumably presented to their students.

(FYI: If students weren't taught the material covered on the Woodcock-Johnson [successfully, one might suppose], then the test used to assess that material would lack for those students "content validity,"[44] thereby calling into question its use in eligibility hearings. (A question, by the way, that's rarely raised, which is curious since teachers' curricula differ vastly across the country). A child's low achievement score, rather than raising concerns about the health and workability of the youngster's brain, might more correctly raise questions about the match between the test materials and/or a teacher's curriculum. Regardless of permutations, a discrepancy between dubious test scores hardly seems reasonable grounds for suggesting a child is mentally or biologically disabled).

Special education's discrepancy formula's lynch pin was (and continues to be) a valid measure of a child's "innate intelligence," the child's potential. Though the Bateman "IQ–Achievement" model was irreparably flawed from its very beginning,[45] and is no longer mandated,[46] the IQ–Achievement discrepancy model lingers even though it is as *invalid* today as it was when first put into practice in the 1970s.[47] Understand, please, that if special education has *no* measure of a child's innate potential, it has *no* valid IQ–Achievement discrepancy model. Despite that possibility, a current student's eligibility for services might hinge on this model's two scores as the field persists in using the defective model.[48] It seems special education doesn't know its own history, or, as has been suggested, it has no qualms about the tentative limb upon which it sits. A knowledgeable, adversarial lawyer could well be the glaring hawk in the trees.

The question has been raised whether IQ should be a component in definitions of LD and dyslexia?[49] "No" is the most valid answer. Special education has long known that ... "[an] IQ test score is not properly interpreted as a measure of a person's potential."[50] Yet, "the LD field has displayed a remarkable propensity to latch onto concepts that are tenuous and controversial. ... The LD field seems addicted to living dangerously."[51]

It's not surprising that most people in the general public, as well as in the medical profession, are unaware that we've never possessed a valid measure of *innate* human intelligence or potential. Few members of either group spend time concerning themselves with such things. They rely on educational psychologists, special education teachers, and school psychologists (and their college professors) as we rely on their various areas of expertise. Thus, they're granted a pardon. We're not so easily exonerated. We know better.

Concepts and definitions of intelligence abound by the dozens, if not by the hundreds. With so many diverse definitions, it is not surprising that we cannot agree on how to measure [it].[52] ... *Standard texts in educational measurement and assessment routinely warn against interpreting IQ scores as measures of intellectual potential.*[53] (Emphases are mine)

[Writes a professor:] "When I first taught a course called 'Intelligence' in the early 1960s, my predecessor kindly gave me his notes which included a list of over 90 different definitions of intelligence that he had found in the literature. I suspect that, if the list has not doubled in the last quarter century, it's at least half again as long."[54]

Intelligence tests tap a small number of environmental experiences rather than measuring a child's innate potential; they should play no role in determining which children should receive special services. If the right cereal box can enhance a youngster's IQ score,[55] we know clearly that an IQ test is a measure of prior learning of skills and knowledge, and "not ... a measure of some underlying native ability."[56]

David Wechsler, author of the most widely used test of intelligence administered to children, has stated clearly that IQ test results are environmentally influenced and, at best, reflect a momentary level of intellectual functioning.[57,58]

If IQ scores are environmentally influenced, what does that tell us about these tests special education and school psychology use in their effort to distinguish children as learning disabled?

[Researchers have] demonstrated that tests of intelligence are basically similar to tests of achievement. Both kinds of tests involve performances depending upon previously acquired information, abilities, and motives. ... Both kinds of tests call upon the results of learning or experience.[59]

IQ tests are achievement tests. They measure what a person has learned, and they are constructed on the assumption that all people to whom a test is given will have had equal opportunity to learn the answers to the questions asked. The assumption is that given equal opportunity, brighter people learn more answers than duller people. The equal-opportunity condition is only approximately met even in the best of circumstances, and it is fragrantly violated when intelligence tests are used with individuals from cultural backgrounds different from the backgrounds of the people whose performance on the test was used to establish its norms or the meaning of its scores.[60]

(FYI: In today's increasingly diverse American population where culture and environment differences shape untold nuances among children from every ethnic background, exclusions from the assumed "normed group" might include most every child.)

The notion that intelligence tests measure innate potential was explicitly rejected in 1975 by a committee of testing experts, appointed by the American Psychological Association's (APA's) Board of Scientific Affairs. APA's Cleary committee declared:

> A distinction is drawn traditionally between intelligence and achievement tests. A naïve statement of the difference is that the intelligence test measures capacity to learn and the achievement test measures what has been learned. But items in all psychological and educational tests measure acquired behavior.

> An attempt to recognize the incongruity of a behavioral measure as a measure of capacity is illustrated by the statement that the intelligence tests contain items that everyone has an equal opportunity to learn. This statement can be dismissed as false. ... There is no merit in maintaining a fiction.[61]

I count as a good friend and honored colleague a psychologist who believes (or once did) that IQ scores provide a sense of what you can expect of a youngster in a classroom, perhaps, life in general. "She's just a 100," he once informed an elementary school teacher who had expressed disappointment in a child's average school work. The implication: "Don't expect much more from the child. She's topped out," my buddy said, as if the child's crankcase could hold no more oil. My friend's offbeat thinking came indirectly from the teachings of a notorious British psychologist, Cyril Burt (1883–1971), who generously provided the field of psychology with his metaphorical "pint jug," a perfect visual image.

In the 1960s, Dr. Burt contended:

> Capacity must obviously limit content. It is impossible for a pint jug to hold more than a pint of milk; and it is equally impossible for a child's educational attainments to rise higher than his educable capacity permits. ... [It's] obviously nonsensical to try to force more education into the child's head than could be fitted in.[62]

Despite nearly universal condemnation of Cyril Burt's perspective that intelligence is fixed, limited in size and scope, unchangeable, represented by IQ, and imprinted indelibly somewhere beneath the dura mater in the cerebral cortex,[63] some school personnel act as though intelligence is measurable and immutable, and that reported IQ scores accurately represent a child's capacity to achieve academically. The belief that IQ scores represent a ceiling above which one cannot rise occasions surprising and humorous interchanges. I remember this one fondly.

> While at the University of Denver, I had just completed a presentation to a group of local public school teachers, the topic primarily classroom behavior management. Customarily, I asked the group for questions. A young woman stood and spoke earnestly, her expressed concerns far afield from the topics I had touched upon.
>
> "I'm worried about one of my students," said the young teacher. "I fear the student is working above his maximum capacity."
>
> (I did flinch.) "I'm not certain I understand," I confessed, the possibility that someone could "work *above* one's maximum capacity" did not compute.
>
> The teacher explained: "The child's getting 'A's in my class yet his intelligence is only average—100 IQ. He should only be making 'C's, don't you think?"
>
> After a brief pause, I answered sincerely, "Your student is very fortunate. He has an exceptionally good teacher."

As you may recall, I received my doctoral training in the glorious southwest desert. Beautiful falls and springs. Hot summers (and soothing, dry 100° midnights), cold winters (relatively), and snow, if any, described as dustings, except in the distant, surrounding mountains where it could be bountiful. I came to the Arizona program with traditional training using standardized tests that included several versions of so-called intelligence assessments. I administered the latter devices according to established protocol, though I'd often calm a jittery youngster or support one with a warm "Do your best. If you need me to repeat something, let me know." Though I might have tweaked standardization, I knew my encouragement, or the restating of an unfamiliar word would *not* alter the child's *innate* aptitude. A mere pat on the back could hardly modify the youngster's biology or genetics. We're talking about innate, i.e., *inherent* potential, after all. Innate means genes, not trips to the local natural history museum or convivial pep talks. Might my tweak have impacted the child's test score? Absolutely. But that speaks to experience, which is why some of us believe an EQ (experience quotient) might be more functional. How does one increase a child's EQ? The same way one increases a child's IQ.

Directed by a departmental professor, I'd often drive into the Arizona desert to a Native American school where I'd administer the test the professor had scheduled. It was mid-spring day, the temps already in the low 90s, the desert in full bloom. The test I used with the school youngster included a section where the boy needed to look at a standardized picture (shown to every child of a similar age) to see if there was something out of tune—like a car with two round and two square wheels. If a child correctly identified the picture's oddity, he'd earn points toward his IQ, a factor that would influence his possible special education eligibility. The picture in question was a black-and-white depiction of a snowy landscape where portions of tree trunks were buried. Though the boy examined the picture's every square millimeter, he failed to see the subtle error. (I had shown the same picture to several advanced college students. *Not one* found the missing component. Does the word "absurd" fit the test picture?) Unable to solve the puzzle in the allotted time, the delightful boy failed to gain points toward his total IQ score. Unfortunately, every point mattered. The higher the score, the greater the chances he'd be eligible for resource help, which would have served him well.

It wasn't until I drove away, traversing the sunbaked desert with its scruffy bushes, its cacti, and long-tailed lizards, that the obvious struck me, perhaps suggesting something about my limited intelligence. My young Native American friend, born and raised on the remote reservation, may never have seen snow in any degree of abundance—a prerequisite to answering the picture-question correctly. I realized how easy it would have been to influence this boy's IQ score simply by talking to him, showing him magazines, taking him to movies, walking with him through a beautiful field of deep snow where he'd see covered trees and buried rocks. He'd have answered that picture-question correctly, or at least have had a better shot at it. The troubling issue was not the one point he missed on that one question. The troubling issue was the principle of that one point. How many other points had he forfeited for lack of experience—not for lack of smarts. If memory serves me, that was the last IQ test I ever administered.

> Error and inaccuracies inherent in the test itself play a major role in final tallies and recommendations.[64]

I always began my university lectures on IQ testing with an interactive discussion on how a child's experience affects his or her IQ test scores. It was the late 1980s, the class of undergraduate educational psychology. After assuring the students that their entire life depended on the answer to the upcoming, singularly critical question, I asked them to jot on paper the answer to "How far is it from Anchorage to Tokyo in miles." (Those weren't the actual cities, but I'll keep the exact ones a secret just in case you're required to take an IQ test and you're asked the same hum-drum question. You'd have an unfair advantage, don't you think, having *experienced* the information before taking the test?)

My question to my students, "How far is it in miles...," elicited a sea of dumb expressions. (The college students might have been more successful had the question asked how many hours rather than miles, but I didn't author the test, an older version you're not likely to find in use today.) I caught sight of one industrious student in the tiered classroom who pulled from his tidy sport coat a pocket atlas. Since I hadn't established any set of rules, he was well within bounds. His good-natured flashing of the atlas earned him appreciative laughs from his classmates, along with a few "That's not fair" from the more competitive of the bunch. He rifled through the pages, checked the distance, and called out his answer. I smiled, allowing the minor transgression. Since I had administered the IQ test many times in previous years, and had access to the answer code, I knew the correct answer—according to the test manual. Lucky me, other-wise I'd have blown that question. Here's what happened. I wrote his answer—taken from the atlas—on the board. Beside it I wrote the answer that was accepted by the IQ test manual. The two answers *didn't match*! I was tickled. The student missed by a quite a few miles the acceptable answer that would have added IQ points to his total score. Said properly, the student's atlas missed the correct answer by a few miles. Or the IQ test manual missed the answer. It didn't really matter. Would we characterize the student as less intelligent because the atlas's authors used a different number than what the IQ test manual allowed? Doubtful.

The lack of rigor in the diagnostic process has led to an accelerated rate of LD identification and LD becoming, by a wide margin, the largest category in special education. Presently, LD accounts for more than 50% of all students with disabilities and more than 5% of all students in school (U.S. Department of Education, 1999). In commenting on the magnitude of the increase in LD prevalence, researchers[65] suggested that, 'Were these epidemic-like figures interpreted by the Center for Disease Control, one might reasonably expect to find a quarantine imposed on the public schools of America.'[66]

Shortly after the IQ–Achievement discrepancy model was introduced in the 1970s, nearly 50% of the states told their local school districts to make the eligibility decision whether or not differences between IQ and achievement were sufficient to qualify as an allowable discrepancy.[67] The states' reluctance to draw a definitive conclusion was understandable since the size of a discrepancy needed to reach justifiable proportions had not been spelled out by (federal) definition. As a result, the discrepancy size used to qualify youngsters for special education services varied from state to state,[68] and the variety of models and procedures for determining a true discrepancy was described as "countless."[69] Subjective eligibility decisions became the norm rather than the exception. As early as 1974, researchers suggested that

> [T]here is little reason to believe and much empirical reason to disbelieve the contention that some arbitrarily weighted function of two variables [a child's achievement and his IQ] will properly define [a learning disability].[70]

The anti-discrepancy model ground swell continued, and inevitably "the discrepancy criterion for LD identification" was seriously challenged,[71] with some anticipating the model's "impending demise."[72] Concerns of many professionals were summed up in 2003, when the then president of the APA, Robert Sternberg, voiced his view that not only did the two instruments used within the discrepancy model assess much of the same, but that special education's discrepancy formulas were error-prone and filled with problematic statistical properties.

The end came, though diehard schools (and riverboat psychologists) continue to rely upon the defective model, one supremely assailable by a competent lawyer. The reauthorized *Individuals with Disabilities Education Act (IDEA)* was signed into law on December 3, 2004, by President George W. Bush. Significant changes from preexisting regulations regarding the identification of specific learning disabilities were communicated to the field of special education. Having felt the heat from reports emanating from both the US House and Senate Committees considering intelligence testing and LD identification, the Office of Special Education and Rehabilitative Services (OSERS) in the US Department of Education made an embarrassing flip-flop. It declared the following:

> With regard to identifying children with specific learning disabilities [SLD] ... states *may not require* the use of a ... discrepancy between intellectual

ability and achievement to determine whether a child has a specific learning disability.[73] (Emphases are mine)

As it was from its very beginning, Sam Kirk's "learning disability" remained at the heart of the eligibility conundrum.

The virtual dissolution of the IQ–Achievement model did not solve special education's problem. It occasioned one. To fill the created eligibility vacuum, a determined group of multidisciplinary professionals often took a needy child's case under the special education table, played with numbers, and decided the child could qualify for benefits under a different category, such as speech and language concerns, or autism spectrum disorder. (Recall Micelle Diament's report: "In some cases, parents admitted that clinicians gave their child an autism diagnosis simply because that label would make [school] services more readily available.")

These rule-benders were *pro-child* with an attitude that said, "I'm gonna get this kid some services." Good for them, and it happened more often than the feds knew. In one study, researchers found that approximately one-third of students said to be "learning-disabled" were clinical cases, "meaning that their eligibility was a discretionary judgment made by a multidisciplinary team (MDT) which was at variance with the statistical (i.e., IQ-discrepancy) information."[74] Under pressure, and learning that the practice was common, the federal office of special education granted an alternative means to diagnose a learning disability, expressly: "An interdisciplinary team may determine that a child *has* a specific learning disability if the child does not achieve *commensurate* with his or her age."[75] (Emphases are mine).

(FYI: With that edict, something mind-boggling happened. Age, as its own variable, was granted enormous power and influence. Think about this, please. "Commensurate with his or her age..." implies that the mere passage of time guarantees universal learning opportunities, that all-six-year olds, because they've lived six years, have had the same experiences or, more so, have been provided exposure to the same experiences. That assumption is a vital component. If the assumption is false, if a child's home or otherwise living situation failed to provide the learning opportunities, then the lack of experience might be what affects a child's school performance. If so, we'd no longer be talking about a child's purported biological learning disability being responsible for the youngster's underachievement, but a deficiency brought on by the child's inadequate life experiences. The two are hardly the same. If we continue to deny the possibility, we might spend months debating the presence of a disability, when what the child needs is months of planned experiences.)

Here's how the alternative works, with variations unique to each valued, dedicated interdisciplinary team.

An interdisciplinary team notices that Child A's work isn't as good as Child B's, C's, D's, E's, or F's work, all the children being the same age and seated in the same teacher's classroom. According to guidelines, Child A can be said to **have** a learning disability because his work doesn't meet the standards set by his same-age peers. Here's part of the problem with that questionable conclusion.

To reach their decision that the different child has a disability, the interdisciplinary team *must ignore* that Child A and the other children don't have the same parents, they don't live in the same house, they don't live in the same neighborhood, they don't have the same privileges, responsibilities, or luxuries, and the children might not even speak the same first language. That they have the same teacher doesn't mean they've been taught the same material. If that's not worrisome enough, consider the following. This alternative diagnostic method that compares children to determine which ones are disabled must assume that all healthy six-year-olds have had the same *opportunities* to achieve the same level of learning. That regardless of background, culture, language skills, parental support, or environmental history, all six-year-olds have had the same chance to visit the Smithsonian. Or the National Air and Space Museum. Or Disneyworld. Or a baseball game. Or a park with swans and sailboats in a pond.

The logic baffles. The child who performs below his same-age classmates may do so for a dozen reasons, where the only disabling feature involved is the rationale used by the interdisciplinary team to draw its conclusion that the child's brain might have a glitch. (Do you wonder how the interdisciplinary team, or anyone for that matter, would prove that the child actually had a learning disability that's said to be responsible for his underachievement? Please see "tautology" below.)

(FYI: In a fair educational world, the interdisciplinary team wouldn't need to force a disability to gain a child services. They'd recognize that a child who struggled to learn was entitled to services (immediately) because the child and his/her teacher would benefit from the extra services. If the rules don't allow that Camelot option, change the rules. We made them; we can alter them.)

Burned by the flawed IQ-Achievement discrepancy model, and accepting that the "child-comparative" approach was hampered by myriad faults, the feds, doggedly determined to accurately verify the presence of a learning disability, a goal that increasingly seemed out of reach, provided special education with yet another diagnostic effort. This relatively new means fell to a strategy known as "Response to Intervention," or "RtI," a methodology that's part of Multi-Tiered System of Supports (MTSS).

An increasing number of states and their school districts have adopted MTSS to both organize and provide services to children. When used as designed, it's a favorable approximation to individualizing curriculum. It's not bullet proof, however. Because of its secondary purpose, it has, in my view, suffered an embarrassing wound to its noble heart.

Let's look at the positives first. Some of us pre-dated the foundation upon which today's RtI is built. We were raised on task analysis, shaping, discrete trials, data collection, single-subject design research, and most essentially using a child's classroom behaviors to alert us to the possibility that our strategies were lacking and were, therefore, in need of correction.

RTI is a framework to provide early, systematic assistance to children having difficulty with their studies. Its hallmarks include early intervention, frequent progress measurement, and increasingly intensive research based instructional strategies. It allows for intervention in the regular classroom before any referral to special education. A major benefit of RTI, according to the Council for Exceptional Children (CEC), is that children do not have to "wait to fail" before they receive help.[76] The above reference to CEC is especially important, a potential anecdote to curriculum *rigor mortis*.

Beyond its many faults, one of the most defective components of the IQ–Achievement discrepancy model related to the delay in providing services until a child was found eligible for those services. Many weeks/ months often passed while debates and further eligibility testing continued. In the meantime, the child languished with a regular education teacher who didn't know what to do. Had the teacher been properly trained, s/he'd not have requested an LD eligibility hearing as the first option. Seeing the student struggling with class assignments, realizing s/he was part of the problem, s/he'd have conferenced with the principal or colleagues to gain instructional suggestions.

Worst of all, the struggling child, after weeks of curriculum suffocation, might be found ineligible for extra assistance, sentencing the youngster to months with the ill-prepared teacher, producing an outcome that benefits no one. Emeritus educator and psychologist Joe Torgesen gave notice:

> The IQ-discrepancy criterion is potentially harmful to students as it results in delaying intervention until the student's achievement is sufficiently low that the discrepancy is achieved. For most students, identification ... occurs at an age when the academic problems are difficult to remediate with the most intense remediation efforts.[77]

MTSS's primary goal is the prevention and remediation of academic and behavioral difficulties through effective classroom instruction that involves close cooperation between general education and special education.[78] Again, when properly employed, MTSS uses a student's responses to interventions as a basis for determining instructional needs.[79] That means that it determines and modifies its strategies by monitoring their effectiveness on student performance. That's the essence of self-regulation where an educator maintains responsibility for his or her own actions rather than assigning fault for underachievement to a child's faulty brain or the categorical designation "learning disability." In my judgment, correctly administered MTSS has much going for it. With one damning exception.

Pointedly, RtI/MTSS has been hijacked. Once again, special education's federal monitors have genuflected to the medical model and its proposition that a child's persistent classroom underachievement is a function of some error *within* the youngster, thus relieving itself and general education of any responsibility. It's the (expletive deleted) LD game again.

> A secondary goal of the RTI models is the provision of useful data that contributes to referral and decision making about students with LDs.[80]

Ugh! Pray tell how so? Here's how so:

> People are identified as LD when they demonstrate low achievement and intractability to *appropriate instruction*.[81,82] "If a child responds poorly to instruction that benefits most students, then this eliminates instructional

quality as an explanation of poor academic growth and instead provides evidence of disability."[83] (Emphases are mine.)

The conclusion absolutely stupefies. Let's first consider appropriate and inappropriate instruction.

- Instruction (as a verb) *is appropriate* for a child when, and only when, it produces the results intended. That's indisputable.
- Instruction (as a verb) *is inappropriate* for a child when it fails to produce the results intended. That's indisputable.
  "Q": What's the purpose of "instruction?"
  "A": To teach a skill or subject.
    Instructing a child is successful only if the child learns what was instructed. If the child fails to learn what was instructed, the instruction failed. The answer: modify the instruction or the instructor.

If instruction fails to produce the desired end, either the desired end has been misjudged by those who make those decisions or the educational instruction used for the child does not match the youngster's readiness skills. Suggesting the child is disabled as an explanation for a lack of success throws out five decades of research supporting the effectiveness of what behavioral psychologists (and many special education resource teachers) know as task analysis and shaping. At the same time, the feds allowed states to opt out of the untenable IQ–Achievement discrepancy model, knowing full well that districts and schools needed a way out of the eligibility conundrum, the Washington rule-makers ducked behind their shadows and offered a new consideration for determining specific LD identification decisions:

> In determining whether a child has a specific learning disability, a local edu-cational agency may use a process which determines if a child responds to *scientific, research-based intervention* as a part of the evaluation procedures. (P.L. 108–446, Section 614(b)(6))[84] (Emphases are mine)

The authoritative-sounding inclusion "scientific, research-based inter-vention" is RtI's LD-eligibility model's backbone. It's the keel that keeps the rickety boat from capsizing. Except it is *all* smoke and mirrors, as fraudulent as a $3 bill. Ballyhooing "scientific, research-based interven-tion" is quintessential theater designed to impress when the purpose behind it isn't impressive. It's the movie set's instant western town that's all facade and nothing else. That's not RtI/MTSS.

RtI/MTSS is a platform from which interventions flow. It's a guiding model, an architect's blueprints laid out on a pickup truck's hood. It's *not* the hammer and nails and saws soon to be in the hands of the carpenters. That the architect did his or her job well doesn't guarantee the carpenter will do the same. As such, RtI/MTSS is only as effective as the strategies used by its practitioners. If you haven't heard, RtI/MTSS is not an easy approach—and it's never claimed to be.[85]

The feds believe there are too many kids on special education's rolls, too many said to be disabled. Great sums of federal and state dollars are flowing in the wrong direction, they'll say. The current feds (and with them many states) have chosen to reduce those numbers one way or another (see: http://www.houstonchronicle.com/denied/). The difficulty the feds face when demanding a reduction in special education's roles centers on how to bring about that cost-saving end. They've chucked (for the most part) the IQ–Achievement discrepancy model, finally admitting to its intractable defects. What's left? Comparing kids of the same age and concluding if one doesn't do as well as the others that the faltering one must be damaged goods. That interpretation requires all involved to wear not just blinders but blindfolds. Leaving us with the proverbial "last man standing," RtI/MTSS. This demanding, empirically based service delivery system has allowed itself to state that if "a child [fails to] respond to scientific, research-based intervention," the child is disabled. That's incredible. Listen up, please. Concluding that a child's lack of classroom achievement is a function of his or her disability invites to the dance what you known as a "tautology," a circular statement that, like a dog chasing its tail, leaves you where you were when the discussion got its start.

> "She's a bright child but her reading is awful. I'm thinking she has a learning disability."
> "Why would you think that?"
> "Because she's a bright child and her reading is awful."
> That's a tautology.
>
> Or, if you prefer,
>
> "She's a bright child but her reading is awful. I'm thinking she has a learning disability."
> "Why would you think that?"
> "For one thing, she's had the same appropriate, scientific, research-based instruction as all the other children."

"But some of those other kids are also having difficulties with their reading. Do you think they all have...?"
"Don't ask."
That's a tautology and then some.

What does the research say about RtI/MTSS's worth at identifying a learning disability? It doesn't say much that's flattering.

[I]t is clear that the inconsistencies in identifying nonresponders in an RTI model are eerily similar to inconsistencies in the IQ–achievement discrepancy method that RTI purports to correct.[86]
At this point, the LD designation based solely on the RTI model would be just as arbitrary.[87]
In fact, "If practitioners across the nation choose different RTI methods of identification, there may be even greater variation in number and type of children identified as having LD than the variation produced by use of IQ–achievement discrepancy."[88]

Much of the rationale for [using RtI] as an LD identification process stems from dissatisfaction [with] the use of the IQ-achievement discrepancy model.[89]

RtI's developers either deluded themselves or they got conned into believing their procedure could do what no one else could. Or, special education's feds are so desperate to find a way to exclude children from special education assistance, they're willing to try most any chicanery to bring that reduction about. RtI, as a diagnostic option, won't accomplish that ill-considered end.

Based on our analysis, RTI has a limited research base that supports its capability to address the issues of over identification, disproportionality, reliability and validity, and consistency in identifying students with LD.[90]

AN INCONCLUSIVE DISABILITY

Stripped of clauses which specify what a learning disability is not, [its] definition is circular, for it states ... that a learning disability is an inability to learn. It is a reflection of the rudimentary state of knowledge in this field that every definition in current use has its focus on what the condition is *not*, leaving what it is unspecified and thus ambiguous.[91] (Emphasis mine)

Thus,

...[W]e cannot describe, except with considerable lack of precision, students called LD. We think that LD can best be defined as "whatever society wants it to be, needs it to be, or will let it be" at any point in time. ... We think researchers have compiled an interesting set of findings on a group of students who are experiencing academic difficulties, who bother their regular classroom teachers and who have been classified by societally sanctioned labelers in order to remove them, to the extent possible, from the regular education mainstream.[92]

...If we continue trying to define learning disabilities by using ill-defined concepts, we will forever be frustrated, for it is an elusive concept. We are being bamboozled. It is as though someone started a great hoax by inventing the term then tempting others to define it. And lo and behold... task forces and others have taken the bait.[93]

Sam Kirk: "Recently, I have used the term 'learning disability' to *describe* a group of children."[94,95] (Emphasis mine)

Dr. Kirk intended his coined term to serve as a useful umbrella, a convenient term under which children with similar characteristics could gather, a nameplate that not only facilitated broad identification, but provided a means to distinguish some children from others. He suggested to the parents at the Chicago conference that the term "learning disability" could be used in place of more distressing labels as "emotionally disturbed," "mentally retarded," or "lazy," designations chosen by some professionals to *describe* underachieving children. Writing about that Chicago day, Kirk recounted: "The parents settled for the more general term 'learning disabilities,' a term that could *cover* a heterogeneous group of children"[96] (Emphasis mine). The informative phrase "could cover a heterogeneous group" tells us what Dr. Kirk had in mind: "LD" was a term to be used as a convenient descriptor of a *group* of children. By wisely including the term "heterogeneous," Kirk cautioned that his coined adjective would do poorly at specifying or differentiating an individual child's curriculum struggles or his or her individual resource needs. His umbrella term, therefore, would provide little *practical* relevance beyond a gathering point as does a flag pole in the center of a city park. If you stand ten kids by the silvery pole, each youngster *described* as "learning disabled," you'll have ten different kids, with ten different curriculum issues, each in need of a different strategy.

Adjectives such as "learning disabled" used to *describe* the children gathered around the flag pole add a quality to a conversation. A "learning disabled" child implies more than the single word "child." Likewise, a "sad" face describes more than just a face. The descriptive terms "sad" and "learning disabled" are known as constructs. Constructs are convenient shorthand terms that make conversation easier but rarely specific enough to convey much useful information.

Constructs, however, are not directly observable. They represent what is observable. We don't see "sad." Instead, we might see a person cry and bury his face in his hands. Based on our own experience with what we've observed, we might assume the individual is feeling sad. There's a problem with that assumption, of course. Happy people, given a set of circumstances, cry and drop their face in their hands. That tells us that constructs do not lend themselves to precise measurement, a problem inherent in the shorthand construct "learning disabled."

Consider the adjective "cold." It, too, is a construct. By itself it speaks only in generalities. Consider describing outside as "cold" without the benefit of useful backup information, like providing the added "30 degrees Fahrenheit" taken from an outdoor thermometer. The numerical temperature reading lets a listener decide if cold is cold, enough to stay hunkered down under goose-feather covers, or don a sweater for 9 holes of golf. "Cold" causes us no problem. We can stick our nose outside and define it for ourselves. Some constructs, however, require more thought.

Recently, I learned of an acquaintance whose daughter had been diagnosed with cerebral palsy. Cerebral palsy is a construct with its own acronym, CP. CP represents the neuromuscular disability's sizable web of symptoms. An individual with CP may exhibit markers so subtle that if you met the person, you'd not notice anything of consequence. Only a trained eye might observe the slight right-leg limp, or the stiffness of the right hand's fingers.

Conversely, CP can be so thoroughly involving that an individual is confined to a wheelchair with insufficient control of muscles needed to speak or exhibit mastery over any limbs. If I were to provide you only the adjective-phrase "a CP child," would you know the individual child's skill sets?

You wouldn't, of course. The acronym, CP, on its own, can paint an entirely misleading picture. There's the drawback of constructs and acronyms. As was the case with "cold," it's helpful to have some data-level information. With "cold," a thermometer's reading, assuming it were accurate, would likely suffice.

With "LD," however, we're left with a construct that has no verified, acceptable backup thermometer. We have, instead, what children do in the context of school and home, their behaviors, specifically their underachievement, itself a construct that is decided subjectively and often by comparison. Recall our Child A who failed to do as well as Child B, C, or D.

A child's observed achievements and underachievement do provide an option where comparing children isn't necessary in order to assign services. We could simply describe child A's behavior, probably what Sam Kirk had in mind, a descriptive narrative that clarified where within the curriculum the child succeeded, and where within the same curriculum the child faltered. A little more work on our part, describing the child's strengths and struggles, but significantly more informative than relying on the adjective "learning disabled."

There's a noted side benefit to this choice if we could convince ourselves to describe in detail the child's academic strengths and weaknesses while concerning ourselves less with disability hunting. The concept of "eligibility" would become irrelevant. Instead, special educators along with regular educators would work with the child where s/he was, the goal being to move the youngster forward along the individualized curriculum.

But the feds changed the proverbial playing field. They established a learning disability as a designated category of special education. The "learning disabled" child, what had been an agreeable, though limited adjective-phrase that was easy to use and non-confrontational, changed colors and became "a child *with* a learning disability," politically more correct, perhaps, but empirically more problematic. In the eyes of many, "learning disabilities" became a noun, a thing, something not unlike the flu, what needed to be diagnosed and treated like other ailments that fell within the medical model. Instead of describing a child as learning disabled as Dr. Kirk proposed, the feds proclaimed that a learning disability was a condition, a flaw *within* the child.

In no time, special education as a field took the impulsive next step, the proverbial slippery slope. It stipulated that "A learning disability can cause a person to have trouble learning and using certain skills,"[97] the adverse consequences of such thinking far-reaching. It gave regular education a free pass, it diverted our attention from factors that were directly involved in a child's achievement struggles, and it took special education down a road it could not successfully navigate, one with a potentially precipitous dead-end.

Know, please, that there's nothing correct about the assertion "a learning disability can cause a person to have trouble learning and using certain skills." The corrupting issue relates to what constitutes a learning disability. A "learning disability," no matter how we massage it, is *not* a biological entity a child has. It lacks the structure necessary to qualify as a "cause" or an "effect."

Today, a half-century after Sam Kirk addressed those troubled parents, "learning disabilities" is as messy a construct as it was when Kirk first coined the term. The sooner special education accepts that, the sooner the field will right itself and make progressive changes in the manner in which it and regular education teachers assist struggling children. The problem that needs rectifying: special education's (and school psychology's) adherence to the misplaced medical model.[98,99]

PNEUMONIA

To help me graphically present the errors made when we suggest that a child's learning disability (or presumed brain damage) is responsible for his underachievement, I'm bequeathing you a favorite cousin who's a little off her game. Follow this critical sequence to its end. Upon arriving, you'll notice that it delivers you, as a teacher or psychologist, precisely where you need to be.

Your favorite cousin tells you she's running a 104 fever, that her body can't decide to sweat or shiver so it does both. She aches, she's weak, and her cough produces a greenish, yellowish yuk. "I have pneumonia. That's *why* I'm feeling so awful," she declares through her misery. Her answer seems sensible. I've charted your cousin's fever, her cough, and her sweating and shivering, which medical doctors and you know as "symptoms." Her entered symptoms are her body's *behaviors*. If those symptoms *weren't* present, pneumonia wouldn't be considered (Box 3.1). Make sense?

Box 3.1   Pneumonia

Symptoms

104 fever. Sweating and shivering. Aching. Weak. Thick wet cough.

Your cousin searched WebMD to learn what walloped her. She entered her symptoms, answered several questions, and learned from a virtual physician that she likely *has* pneumonia and that's the *cause* of her woes. Though the advice sounds right, the virtual doc's answer is *wrong*, the point significant as we consider *all* educationally framed disabilities.

WebMD's virtual docs are confident that typical visitors don't hold degrees in respiratory infections or internal medicine. They, therefore, select their words carefully. In your cousin's case, they chose the familiar term "pneumonia" when your cousin described her ills. I'll insert pneumonia under our boxes dual "cause/has" column (Box 3.2).

Box 3.2   Pneumonia

Cause/Has	*Symptoms*
Pneumonia	Fever. Sweating and Shivering. Aching. Weak. Thick wet cough. Yuk

---

Here's the rub.

- **First**, pneumonia is *not* the cause of your cousin's symptoms.
- **Second**, pneumonia is *not* something to have.
- **Third**, "pneumonia" *is* merely an accessible, useful, shorthand term, what we've called a "construct," a word that makes conversation easier, though invariably void of details.
- **Fourth**, the cause(s) of your cousin's symptoms remains (temporarily) unknown, hence the added question mark under the "cause" column in the following box. While the symptoms have remained the same, I've repositioned "pneumonia" where it belongs—under the important new heading that I've named "convenient construct" (Box 3.3).

Box 3.3   Pneumonia

Cause	*Convenient Construct*	*Symptoms*
?	Pneumonia	Fever. Sweating and Shivering. Aching. Weak. Thick wet cough. Yuk

- **Fifth,** medical doctors *don't* treat pneumonia. That's a critical point. Medical docs treat the fever, the cough, the yuk—*and* what's thought to be at the root of the fever, the cough, and the yuk. Think about that last statement. Medical docs treat the symptoms *and* what's *contributing* to those symptoms. "Contributing" is the essential word, particularly when we look at learning disabilities. In pneumonia's case, *those* contributors happen to be tiny critters that have invaded your cousin's body, critters that are measurable[100] and thus verifiable *or* refutable, both possible outcomes essential components of the scientific model.

What does your cousin have? She has either a bacterial or viral infection known by the very rude, cumbersome names *Pneumocystis jiroveci, streptococcus,* Group B, *Mycoplasma pneumoniae.* Your cousin's doctor treats symptoms and the verifiable, strangely named bugs that have produced the respiratory infection and the rest of her ills. "Pneumonia" is merely *window dressing,* that earlier mentioned shorthand construct, a word that has no role in any technical discussion. Look closely. Our corrected box reads as follows (Box 3.4).

Box 3.4   Pneumonia

Cause	*Convenient Construct*	*Symptoms*	*Intervention*
Pneumocystis jiroveci, Mycoplasma pneumoniae	Pneumonia	Fever. Sweating and Shivering. Aching. Weak. Cough. Yuk	Multiple

But the box needs one more adjustment. Once your cousin begins treatment (if not before), the approachable term "pneumonia" is no longer needed. Initially, it was used for your cousin's benefit, and for the benefit of her commiserating family who gathered around and wanted to know what was wrong with their favorite lady. Better the family heard "pneumonia" from the physician than "*Pneumocystis jiroveci, streptococcus,* Group B, *Mycoplasma pneumoniae.*" "Pneumonia," however, serves little purpose for the medical staff that might await a lab report to verify the bugs' presence. The final box, properly without the construct "pneumonia," looks like this (Box 3.5).

Box 3.5 Pneumonia

Cause	Symptoms	Intervention
Pneumocystis jiroveci, Mycoplasma pneumoniae	Fever. Sweating and Shivering. Aching. Weak. Cough. Yuk	Multiple

We have our cause, our symptoms, and our soon to be revealed medical strategies to deal with both. That's the medical model. As it refers to *Pneumocystis jiroveci, streptococcus,* it works fine, and your likeable cousin, barring unforeseen circumstances, like stumbling over her newly rescued kitten, will be up and around shortly.

Let's apply the same sequence to special education's use of the model. Interesting problems abound.

LEARNING DISABILITY

Nothing of consequence changes by replacing "pneumonia" with the term "Learning Disability." As with pneumonia, we start with the "symptoms" that the child exhibits in his or her classroom. Let's name the general problem *underachievement*. (Staff will need to operationalize the term at the data level so we know precisely what the shorthand construct "underachievement" represents. I'll approximate this "data level" when we look at "dyslexia.") Realize that if the child in question achieved in the classroom as expected, a learning disability would not be suspected or suggested. With LD, our initial box looks like this (Box 3.6).

Box 3.6 Learning disabilities

Cause	Convenient Construct	Behaviors••	Intervention
Unknown	?	Underachievement	?

(•• Notice I've replaced "symptoms" with the term "behaviors," what the child is observed to do in the classroom. "Symptoms" is a medical term that with scarce exception doesn't belong in any discussion regarding a child's classroom achievement or underachievement.)

Next, we'll consider the suggestion that an LD is responsible for your child's achievement woes. Again, it has been stated that "[a] learning disability [LD] can *cause* a person to have trouble learning and using certain skills" (Box 3.7).[101]

Box 3.7   Learning disabilities

Cause/Has••	Convenient Construct	Behaviors	Intervention
Learning Disability		Underachievement	

Asserting LD as the "cause" for your child's underachievement is *not* a valid claim for several reasons. Foremost, Sam Kirk did not intend his term to be used in that manner. He spoke of an LD as a shorthand construct that he used to *describe* children, not a condition or factor that could *cause* or explain an outcome. Any of us can play with words to satisfy our personal whims, but the meaning of the term "learning disability" as Sam Kirk intended, remains. Further, even as a descriptive construct, "learning disability" is neither measurable nor diagnosable. We don't see a learning disability, and we have no educational litmus test that can accurately verify or deny its presence or absence. Accordingly, I've moved "learning disability" from "Cause" and inserted it under "Convenient Construct" where it accurately serves as Sam Kirk's umbrella term. "Cause" as it pertains to the child's underachievement, remains unknown (Box 3.8).

Box 3.8   Learning disabilities

Cause	Convenient Construct	Behaviors	Intervention
?	Learning Disability	Underachievement	?

CAUSE

Many in special education have long pointed to a malfunctioning brain as the explanation or cause for a child's scholastic underachievement. A child's brain has always been the *go-to* answer when legitimate answers to account for observations are hard to come by. From LD's inception, special education has pointed to a malfunctioning brain when explaining a child's inadequate classroom performance; for example:

- Maturational lag in general neurological development[102]
- Failure of the brain to establish cerebral dominance[103]
- Failure to achieve certain states of neurological development[104]

Special education (and the medical profession) chose to define LD as a disorder with a biological base, an easy decision to make.

> The designation of learning disabled appeared to be an almost ideal solution: it implied no stigma on either the child or his parents, carried no racial overtones, and suggested an ailment that was the metaphorical corollary of an electronic malfunction—faulty wiring in the cortex or central nervous system. The child wasn't sick; he was simply disabled.[105]

Though the biological choice is a *safe* answer, meaning the hypothesized faulty wiring and/or a weakened set of synapses *can't be* verified *or* refuted, I've abided by special education's expedient decision, and listed "brain damage" as a possible cause for a child's classroom underachievement. LD remains as a construct, and the child's problem continues to be his or her underachievement (Box 3.9).

Box 3.9   Learning disabilities

Cause	Convenient Construct	Behaviors	Intervention
Brain damage	Learning disability	Underachievement	?

(**FYI**: "Whenever a disruptive classroom behavior pattern was observed, it was interpreted to reflect an underlying biological damage that had impaired a child's brain,"[106] which would be called "minimal brain damage" (MBD).[107,108] In the 1960s, "minimal brain damage" would be further amended to "minimal brain dysfunction syndrome,"[109] the term "damage" being removed because no recognized organic damage could be found.[110])

The decision to posit brain damage as the cause for a child's achievement struggles was, and has always been, a disastrous choice. It sanctioned the option to ignore the relationship between general education's systemic inadequacies and children's classroom struggles. If a child failed to reach standards set for all children of the same age, if he or she scored lower on reading achievement tests (in comparison to others), if he or she stubbornly reversed letters, persistently miscalculated math problems, or wrote cursive that resembled chicken scratch, then the child must somehow be burdened by a biological error centered in his or her brain. The classroom was *not* a contributor. The teachers were *not* a contributor. The curriculum was *not* a contributor. The child's interest or motivation, home support, healthy breakfast (or its absence) were *not* contributors. The cause was biological—a physiological error within the child.[111] Simple enough, and extraordinarily shortsighted.

We *can* hypothesize that a brain anomaly is responsible for a child's observed and documented academic struggles. Special education teachers and school psychologists who work with exception kids know that such a connection sometimes exists, though the actual cerebral damage is inferred (and rarely confirmed). But it would be entirely *wrong* to suggest that a malfunctioning brain *is responsible for a learning disability*. "Learning disability" is simply a generated name, Sam Kirk's convenient construct, one that represents what a child does. Standing alone, as pointed out, it has no physical structure.

Only a child's classroom underachievement, his or her actual behavior, is measurable and thus possibly affected by the brain's blemish, though such underachievement is more likely related to any number of non-organic variables within the child's active environment.

How best to use the term "learning disability?" Many bright children struggle with reading and/or mathematics. Does the term "learning disability" fit such situations? *Only* if used as a descriptive adjective, that is, "he's learning disabled," a statement that tells us very little of importance about a youngster. When used as a noun, as an explanation, that the child reads poorly *because* she *has* a learning disability, we've committed a serious methodological (and tautological) error. How do we know she has an LD? Because she struggles with reading. We have *no* verifiable, brain-based cause for any child's specific classroom underachievement involving our iconic 3Rs. Is brain damage possible? Certainly. Does it matter? *Only if it's reversible*. But here's what *does* matter. If we accept the constructs LD or MBD or dyslexia as *causes* for a child's underachievement, the child's teacher and school won't need to examine what's happening in the classroom. Overlooking classroom mechanics, i.e., how a teacher teaches, what curriculum the teacher uses, is a major error, if not an ethical oversight. Finally, with respect to the construct "learning disabilities" and our box, two pieces of house cleaning remain. When considering strategies, it matters not if we classify a child disabled, disordered, or simply a different learner. Since the construct "learning disability" fails to specify what strategies will assist the child, the construct, perhaps beyond providing the child special education's services, becomes a superfluous term. Accordingly, I've removed "learning disability" from the box, the action having *no* bearing on the child. Additionally, since no biological cause for any child's underachievement is verifiable, it, too, needs to be removed from the box. Leaving us exactly where we need to be:

With a child who sometimes succeeds and sometimes doesn't succeed with his/her assigned curriculum.

With trained staff who will task and error analyze the child's achievement strengths and weaknesses.

With all the strategies that general and special education have developed to help the child improve (Box 3.10).

Box 3.10 Learning disabilities	
Behaviors	*Intervention*
A child's successful and unsuccessful achievement	Multiple educational strategies

Dyslexia

The terms "dyslexia," "dyscalculia," and "dysgraphia" represent reading, writing, and arithmetic—with the added implication that a child who fails to read, write, and do math as well as others, or as well as his or her IQ score predicts, *has* a learning disability. To restate the obvious, the comparative performance between children and the use of IQ tests are invalid operations with which to suggest, much less authenticate, a learning disability.

You can run any of the "Ds" through the previous boxes. The outcome will be the same. Let's do "dyslexia." It's gaining a lot of attention once again: "Parents Call for Support On Dyslexic Students."[112] Actually, "dyslexia" is *not* gaining the attention. Children's reading struggles are at the heart of the parents' demands. Remember, we don't see "dyslexia." We do see children struggle with school achievement, reading specifically. The point may seem trivial. It's not. As always, we start with a child's behaviors, what we observe the child doing in the classroom. We'll need to know specifics, not just what the child struggles with, but what he or she succeeds at reliably. More on that latter point in Chap. 5. Documenting a child's strengths is extremely important when developing strategies. (See below, please.) For brevity, let's stipulate that a child exhibits letter reversals, word omissions, and sound-symbol difficulties (Box 3.11).

Box 3.11   Dyslexia

Behaviors••	*Strategies*
Letter reversals, word omissions, sound-symbol difficulties	?

Let's further suggest that the child exhibits those behaviors *because* he or she *has* "dyslexia" (Box 3.12).

Box 3.12   Dyslexia

Cause/Has••	*Convenient Construct*	*Behaviors*	*Strategies*
Dyslexia		Letter reversals, word omissions, sound-symbol difficulties	

That tautological conclusion would be incorrect, of course. The child reverses his letters because he has dyslexia. How do you know he has dyslexia? Because he reverses his letters. "Dyslexia" is a shorthand term that represents the related behaviors a child exhibits. It, like learning disabilities, is a construct, neither a cause nor an effect. The "effect" would be the child's behavior, the child's reading difficulties. Thus, we must place the term "dyslexia" where it belongs, under the "Convenient Construct" heading. That leaves "cause" unknown (Box 3.13).

Box 3.13   Dyslexia

Cause	Convenient Construct	Behaviors	Strategies
?	Dyslexia	Letter reversals, word omissions, sound-symbol difficulties	?

Predictably, the medical model suggests that "dyslexia" is caused by an error within the brain. "Dyslexia is due to a defect in the brain's processing of graphic symbols" (Box 3.14).[113]

Box 3.14   Dyslexia

Cause	Convenient Construct	Behaviors	Strategies
Brain error	Dyslexia	Letter reversals, word omissions, sound-symbol difficulties	?

The brain-defect assertion is both misleading and wrong. The fault in the brain, if it exists, and if it were proven to be *specific* to a child's decoding skills, would be responsible for the child's letter reversals, word omissions, and sound-symbol difficulties, not the label, "dyslexia."

(FYI: From a practical point of view, the term "dyslexia" is a distraction. In this instance, if we intend to help the child, we need to know the youngster's skill sets: the particular letters reversed, the words omitted, the troubling sound-symbols, as well as the particular letters, words, and sound-symbols the child has mastered. We often focus only on the child's deficits. If we wish to help the child improve his/her reading skills, it's wise to remember that we don't help a child ascend a challenging mountain knowing only what s/he "can't" do.)

Though the proposed brain anomaly provides a teacher or parent with a possible explanation for a child's reading struggles, one that perhaps eases their anxieties, the answer may be incorrect.[114] While the issue will be deliberated, with some authorities at Duke and Yale suggesting that "the term 'dyslexia' be abandoned altogether because it is unscientific and lacks meaning,"[115] Sally Shaywitz has turned our attention away from that tiresome debate, the construct "dyslexia" always the elusive component. Dr. Shaywitz has suggested that a good reading program may assist the "dyslexic" brain repair itself. Whether that remarkable claim is valid or not is secondary to what Dr. Shaywitz asserts is responsible for the brain's cellular change, that being a "year-long reading program that consisted of a very good set of reading strategies."

(FYI: I think we'd like all kids to experience in some fashion a year-long reading program that consisted of a very good set of reading strategies from the first day of school.)

Dr. Shaywitz's observation does allow us to speculate that for some children who missed out on such stellar instruction, letter reversals, word omissions, and sound-symbol difficulties may have had their *start* with a *poor set* of reading strategies, that inadequate instruction, rather than the child's unique brain, might have *contributed* to the child's reading underachievement. Let us adjust the box (Box 3.15).

Box 3.15 Dyslexia

Contributor	Behaviors	Strategies
Inadequate reading instruction	Letter reversals, word omissions, sound-symbol difficulties	?

Since inadequate reading instruction is speculation, we'll remove the supposition as a possible, though non-verifiable past event, leaving us with a box that tells us what we have, and leaves open what we need to do to help the child (Box 3.16).

Box 3.16   Dyslexia

Behaviors	Strategies
Letter reversals, word omissions, sound-symbol difficulties	?

Notice that we've come full circle with our school child's classroom achievement challenges, struggles that were no doubt observed many months earlier. We've wasted precious time focusing on labels requiring professionals to dillydally with federal, state, and a district's paper requirement where what was needed months earlier was their expertise (what Daniel Hallahan insists is "intensive individualized instruction")[116] delivered to a waiting child, instruction that targeted specific learning needs. With letter reversals, word omissions, sound-symbol difficulties, the strategy recommendation will not come as a surprise (Box 3.17).

Box 3.17   Dyslexia

Behaviors	Strategies
Letter reversals, word omissions, sound-symbol difficulties	Treatment should be directed to the specific learning problems of the affected individual. The usual course is to modify teaching methods and the educational environment to meet the specific needs of the individual.[a]

[a]http://www.medicinenet.com/script/main/art.asp?articlekey=3138

We would say the same whether we're talking about a child who demonstrated problems with writing or mathematics, or with any other subject area or curricular assignment that create problems for kids. The constructs that we use to describe the child, whether LD or dyslexic, dysgraphic or dyscalculic, are irrelevant to our strategies. Indeed, the same can be said for purported biological contributors such as brain damage that are not reversible.

> From an educational point of view, the cause of a condition rarely is relevant for remediation. To know the etiology does not change the educational program. [Good] teachers use a developmental curriculum, starting where a child is and helping the child move the developmental ladder step by step. —Sam Kirk[117]

For self-regulating professionals, those who maintain responsibility for a child's success, strategies matter the most.

EPILOGUE

Children said to be learning disabled will be whatever people choose them to be. Naming them as such satisfies us, perhaps, but it does little that's practical for the child. Corralling LD, and providing struggling children with the best intervention, is not going to happen, not if we continue to hold the traditional definition espoused by The National Joint Committee on Learning Disabilities (NJCLD):

> Learning disorders and disabilities are "presumed ... due to [caused by] a central nervous system dysfunction."[118]

What needs to be discovered to assist any child won't be found in either a child's brain or with whatever else we propose is wrong with the youngster. Special education will never rescue itself from its own quicksand until it relinquishes the belief that a learning disability is a real, identifiable biological condition that's caused by another real identifiable biological condition.

> I have felt for some time that labels we give children are satisfying to us, but of little help to the child himself. We seem to be satisfied if we can give a technical name to a condition. This gives us the satisfaction of closure. We think we know the answers if we can give the child a name or a label—brain injured, schizophrenic, autistic, mentally retarded, aphasi[c], etc. ... The terms cerebral palsy, brain injured, mentally retarded, aphasic, etc. are not classification terms. They are not diagnostic, if by diagnosis we mean an assessment of the child in such a way that leads us to some form of treatment, management, or remediation. —Sam Kirk[119]

Beyond the fact that the stubborn concept of a learning disability has outlived its usefulness, its existence permits general education to avoid monitoring its own fallible methods, its failures in structure and delivery often evident within days of a child's first visit to school.

> One wonders if real progress will not come from disentangling children from this huge conglomerate mass, rigorously specifying the nature of their difficulties, and systematically exploring educational interventions?[120]

To the extent that we permit crafted disabilities to cover regular education's systemic inadequacies, we're complicit in maintaining a medical model fiction that we initiated decades ago. It's the same fiction that we maintain today either by choice or by default, the latter because we refuse to openly challenge the objectionable status quo. Not everyone has chosen to look the other way, however. Many school psych buddies who work with kids retrained themselves and put away their WISC kits years ago. Many honored special education school-based engineers focus entirely on the child, not the label some committee has sanctioned. Change is possible, but not by its own impetus.

I want to share this with you. I was most fortunate to have been involved.

For a brief period of time many years ago, a special education director I knew and admired worked out a deal with the state of Colorado to allow special education teachers to serve all children (in his district) without the need for LD eligibility. The services were provided to the children based on identified need with no loss of funds to the district. The children were pleased, the parents were pleased, the special ed teachers were pleased, and I believe many in Colorado's State Department were pleased. And the earth, without a hitch, continued to turn on its axis.

[L]earning disabilities today satisfies so many varied personal and professional agendas that it has become impossibly murky. It has evolved to represent a vague construct complicated by substantial heterogeneity.[121] It represents so many idiosyncrasies that it provides no categorical value. Each learning disabled individual is his or her own star, making the term useless when applied to an entire group. Because each child said to be learning disabled is unique, [because] each shows a different combination and severity of problem. ... Samuel Kirk's "learning disability" no longer says anything meaningful about any of them. It is time we get past the attempt at a consensus definition and onto the children who need assistance.[122]

NOTES

1. Rosenthal, B.M. & Barned-Smith, St. J.B. (December 12, 2016). Angry parents in Houston and Dallas turn out at forums, demanding end to special education target. *Houston Chronicle*. Retrieved from http://www. houstonchronicle.com/news/houston-texas/houston/article/Angry-parents-in-Houston-and-Dallas-turn-out-at-10792247.php?t=f373f5bc6 f438d9cbb&cmpid=twitter-premium.

2. Martin, R. (1992, July/August). Problems with severe discrepancy formulas. *LDA/Newsbriefs*, 3.
3. Martin. E.W., Martin, R., & Terman, D.L. (Spring, 1996). The Legislative and Litigation History of Special Education. *The Future of Children.* See: http://wwfinductionmodules-resources.wiki.educ.msu.edu/file/view/History+of+Special+Education.pdf.
4. Henley, M., Ramsey, R.S., & Algozzine, R. (1993). *Characteristics of and strategies for teaching students with mild disabilities.* (p. 5). Boston: Allyn & Bacon.
5. Henley, M., Ramsey, R.S., & Algozzine, R. (1993). (p. 5).
6. Heller, W.H., Holtzman, W.H., & Messick, S. (1982). Placement in special education: Historical developments and current procedures. In Kirby A. Heller, Wayne H. Holtzman, & Samuel Messick (Eds.), *Placing children in special education: A strategy for equity* (p. 32). Washington, DC: National Academic Press.
7. Smith, D.D., & Luckasson, R. (1992). *Introduction to special education: teaching in an age of challenge.* (pp. 20–21). Boston: Allyn & Bacon.
8. West, J. (January 25, 2000.) Back to school on civil rights: Advancing the federal commitment to leave no child behind. *National Council on Disability.* Retrieved from https://eric.ed.gov/?id=ED438632.
9. Schrag, P., & Divoky, D. (1975). *The myth of the hyperactive child & other means of child control.* (pp. 48–50). New York: Pantheon Books.
10. Schrag, P., & Divoky, D. (1975), (pp. 48–50).
11. Samuels, C. (January 29, 2015) Free Online Course for Teachers, Coaches to Focus on 'Learning Differences'. *Education Week* blog. Retrieved from http://blogs.edweek.org/edweek/speced/2015/01/free_online_course_for_teacher.html.
12. Baucom. J. (April 12, 2013). Learning disability movement turns 50. *Washington Post.* Retrieved from https://www.washingtonpost.com/news/answer-sheet/wp/2013/04/12/learning-disabilities-movement-turns-50/?utm_term=.79479dc6cb83.
13. Hallahan, D.P., Lloyd, J.W., Kauffman, J.M., Weiss, M.P., & Martinez, E.A. (2005) *Learning disabilities foundation.* Boston: Allyn & Bacon/Longman.
14. Schrag, P., & Divoky, D. (1975). (p.50).
15. Hallahan, D.H. & Mercer, C.D. (2001). Learning disabilities: Historical perspective. Retrieved from http://ldsummit.air.org/download/Hallahan%20Final%202008-10-01.pdf.
16. Smith, R.M. & Neisworth, J.T. (1975). *The exceptional child: A functional approach.* New York: McGraw-Hill.
17. Schrag, P., & Divoky, D. (1975). (p. 35).
18. Ysseldyke, J.E., Algozzine, B., & Thurlow, M.L. (1992). *Critical issues in special education.* (p. 350). Boston: Houghton Mifflin Company.

19. Kavale, K.A., & Forness, S.R. (2000). History, rhetoric, and reality: Analysis of the inclusion debate. *Remedial and Special Education, 33,* 130–137.
20. Danielson, L.C., & Bauer, J.N. (1978). A formula-based classification of learning disabled children: An examination of the issues. *Journal of Learning Disabilities, 11,* 163–176.
21. Winters, M.A. & Greene, J.P. Debunking a special education myth. *EducationNext.* Spring 2007, Vol. 7, No. 2 http://educationnext.org/debunking-a-special-education-myth/.
22. Mash, E.J., & Wolfe, D.A. (2013). *Abnormal Child Psychology* (p. 331). Belmont, CA: Wadsworth.
23. Batstra L., Hadders-Algra M., Nieweg E., VanTol D., Pijl S.J., Frances A. Childhood emotional and behavioral problems: reducing overdiagnosis without risking undertreatment. Dev Med Child Neurol. 2012; 54: 492–494.
24. Frances, A. (2012) "America's False Autism Epidemic," *New York Post,* April 23, 2012. Reprinted with permission in, Autism (2014). Introducing Issues with Opposing Viewpoints. Lauri. S. Scherer, Ed. Farmington Hills, MI: Greenhaven Press. p. 50.
25. Shattuck, P. (2005–2017). Autism cases on the rise: Reason for increase a mystery. *Web.com.* Retrieved from http://www.webmd.com/brain/autism/searching-for-answers/autism-rise.
26. Reynolds, C.R. (1985). Critical measurement issues in learning disabilities. *Journal of Special Education, 18,* 451–475.
27. Martin, R. (1992 July/August), (p. 3).
28. Anonymous. (Undated). Calculating the 'excess cost' of educating children with disabilities. *newamerica.org.* Retrieved from http://febp.newamerica.net/background-analysis/individuals-disabilities-education-act-funding-distribution.
29. Chambers, J.G., Parrish, T.B., & Harr, Jenifer J. (September, 2002). What Are We Spending on Special Education Services in the United States, 1999-2000? *Eric.ed.gov. Report. Special Education Expenditure Project (SEEP).* Retrieved from http://eric.ed.gov/?id=ED471888.
30. Beales, J.R. (1993). Special education: Expenditures and obligations, *Reason Foundation,* Policy Study No. 161, (p. 13).
31. Dan Goldberg. (July 6, 2010). "N.J. School Districts Avoid Cuts in Special Education in Budget Crisis," *Star-Ledger.* Newark, NJ.
32. McCann, C. (2014) Federal funding for students with disabilities. *New America Education Policy Brief.* Retrieved from http://files.eric.ed.gov/fulltext/ED556326.pdf.
33. Reeve, R.E., & Kauffman, J.M. Learning disabilities. In V.B. Van Hassett, P.S. Strain, & M. Hersen (Eds.), *Handbook of developmental and physical*

disabilities. New York: Plenum. Reported in Patton, J.R., Payne, J.S., Kauffman, J.M, Brown, G.B., & Payne, R.A. (1987). *Exceptional children in focus.* (p. 13). Columbus: Merrill Publishing Company.

34. Cruickshank, W.M. (1972). Some issues facing the field of learning disabilities. *Journal of Learning Disabilities, 5,* 380–388.

35. Kavale & Forness, 2000.

36. Willson, V.L. (May, 1996), 16:53:55-0500 (*Psychoeducationallistserv*).

37. Anonymous. Introduction to learning disabilities. *naset.org.* Retrieved from http://www.naset.org/2522.0.html.

38. Bateman, B. (1992). Learning Disabilities: The changing landscape. *Journal of Learning Disabilities, 25,* 29–36.

39. Author anonymous. (2007). What is the IQ-achievement discrepancy model? *Ideapartnershipo.org.* Retrieved from http://www.ideapartnership. org/documents/IQ-RTI.pdf.

40. Bateman, B.D. (1965). An educational view of a diagnostic approach to learning disabilities. In J. Hellmuth (Ed.), *Learning disorders* (Vol. 1, pp. 219–239). Seattle, WA: Special Child Publications.

41. Chalfant, J.C., & King, F.S. (1976). An approach to operationalizing the definition of learning disabilities. *Journal of Learning Disabilities, 9,* 228–243; Frankenberger, W., & Fronzaglio, K. (1991). A review of states' criteria and procedures for identifying children with learning disabilities. *Journal of Learning Disabilities, 24,* 495–500;Mercer, C.D., Jordan, L., Allsopp, D.H., & Mercer, A.R. (1996). Learning disabilities definitions and criteria used by state education departments. *Journal of Learning Disabilities, 19,* 217–232.

42. Note: Construct validity is the extent to which a test measures the concept or construct that it is intended to measure. See: http://www. psychologyandsociety.com/constructvalidity.html.

43. Note: Content validity refers to how accurately an assessment or measurement tool taps into the various aspects of the specific construct in question. In other words, do the questions really assess the construct in question, or are the responses by the person answering the questions influenced by other factors? See: http://education-portal.com/academy/lesson/content-validity-definition-index-examples.html.

44. An educational test with strong content validity will represent the subjects taught to students, rather than asking unrelated questions. See: https://explorable.com/content-validity.

45. Sussan, T.A., Greenwald, S.J., &, Wesler, J.M. (March 25, 2015). How does the school decide if my child has a specific learning disability? Retrieved from http://www.special-ed-law.com/blog/item/64-how-does-the-school-decide-if-my-child-has-a-specific-learning-disability.

46. Greer, M. (April 2005). An alternative idea. *apa.org*. Retrieved from http://www.apa.org/monitor/apr05/idea.aspx.
47. Sussan, T.A., Greenwald, S.J., &, Wesler, J.M. (March 25, 2015).
48. Sussan, T.A., Greenwald, S.J., &, Wesler, J.M. (March 25, 2015).
49. Siegel, L.S. (1990). IQ and learning disabilities: R.I.P. In H.L. Swanson & B. Keogh (Eds.), *Learning disabilities: Theoretical and research issues* (pp. 111–128). Hillsdale, NJ: Erlbaum.
50. Stanovich, K.E. (1991b). Discrepancy definitions of reading disability: Has intelligence led us astray? *Reading Research Quarterly, 26,* 7–29, p. 10.
51. Stanovich, K.E. (1989). Has the learning disabilities field lost its intelligence? *Journal of Learning Disabilities, 22,* 487–492, p. 487.
52. Wesman, A.G. (1968). Intelligence testing. *American Psychologist, 23.*
53. Stanovich, K.E. (1991). Conceptual and empirical problems with discrepancy definitions of reading disability. Learning Disability Quarterly, 14, 269–280.
54. Lezak, M.D. (1988). IQ: R.I.P. Journal of Clinical and Experimental Neuropsychology, 10.
55. Begley, S. (1996, May 6). The IQ Puzzle. *Newsweek,* p. 70.
56. Albee, G.W. (1980). Open letter in response to D.O. Hebb. *American Psychologist, 35,* 386–387.
57. Wechsler, D. (1974). Manual for the Wechsler Intelligence Scale for Children-Revised. New York: Psychological Corp.
58. Baldwin, R.S. & Vaughn, S. (1988). Why Siegel's arguments are irrelevant to the definitions of learning disabilities. *Journal of Learning Disabilities, 22,* 513.
59. Hunt, J. McV., & Kirk, G.E. ((1971). Social aspects of intelligence: Evidence and issues. In Robert Cancro (Ed.). *Intelligence: genetic and environmental influences.* New York: Grune & Stratton. See also: Humphreys, L.G. (1962). The nature and organization of human abilities. In M. Katz (Ed.), *The 19th Yearbook of the National Council on Measurement in Education.* Ames, Iowa.
60. Hobbs, Nicholas (1975). *The futures of children: Categories, labels, and their consequences.* Jossey-Bass: San Francisco, CA. p. 47.
61. Eysenck, H.J., & Kamin, L. (1981). *The intelligence controversy.* New York: John Wiley & Sons.
62. Eysenck, H.J. & Kamin, L. (1981). (p. 94).
63. Kaufman, A.S. (1990). *Assessing adolescent and adult intelligence.* Boston: Allyn & Bacon. p. 60.
64. Kaufman, S.B. (JUL 7, 2013) IQ tests hurt kids, schools–and don't measure intelligence. *Salop.com.* Retrieved from http://www.salon.com/2013/07/07/iq_tests_hurt_kids_schools_and_dont_measure_intelligence/.

65. Macmillan, D.L., Gresham, F.M., Siperstein, G.N., & Bocian, K.M. (1996). The labyrinth of IDEA: School decisions on referred students with subaverage general intelligence. *American Journal on Mental Retardation, 101,* 161–174.
66. Lerner, J. W. (Ed.) (2002). Learning disabilities. *Idaamerica.org.* Retrieved from https://ldaamerica.org/wp-content/uploads/2013/09/ld-journal-spring-2002pdf.
67. Henley, M., Ramsey, R.S., & Algozzine, R. (1993).
68. Hunt, N. & Marshall, K. (1994) *Exceptional Children and Youth.* Boston: Houghton Mifflin.
69. Reynolds, C.R. (1990). Conceptual and technical problems in learning disability diagnosis. In C.R. Reynolds, & R.W. Kamphaus, (Eds.), *Handbook of psychological and educational assessment of children: Intelligence and achievement.* (p. 574). New York: Guilford.
70. Divoky, D. (1974).
71. Kavale, K. http://www.ldaofky.org.
72. Aaron, P.G. (1997). The impending demise of the discrepancy formula. *Review of Educational Research, 67,* 461–502.
73. Myers, C. (2011). Guidelines for identifying students with specific learning disabilities. *cde.state.co.us.* Retrieved from https://www.cde.state.co.us/sites/default/files/documents/cdesped/download/pdf/sld_guidelines.pdf.
74. Shepard, L.A., & Smith, M.L. (1983). An evaluation of the identification of learning disabled students in Colorado. *Learning Disability Quarterly, 6,* 115–127.
75. Chalfant, J.C., & King, F.S. (1976).
76. Lohman, J. (January 17, 2007). *Response to Intervention Plans.* OLR Research Report.
77. Torgesen, J.K. (2004). Lessons Learned From the Last 20 Years of Research on Interventions for Students who Experience Difficulty Learning to Read. In McCardle, P. & Chhabra, V. (Eds.) The voice of evidence in reading research. Baltimore: Brookes Publishing.
78. Fletcher, J.M. & Vaughn, S. (2009). Response to Intervention: Preventing and Remediating Academic Difficulties. *Child Development Perspectives. Vol 3,* Number 1, pp. 30–37.
79. East, B. (2006). Myths about response to intervention implementation. *National Association of State Directors of Special Education.* Retrieved from http://www.rtinetwork.org/learn/what/mythsaboutrti.
80. Fletcher, J.M. & Vaughn, S. (2009).
81. Fuchs, L.S., & Fuchs, D. (1998). Treatment validity: A unifying concept for reconceptualizing the identification of learning disabilities. *Learning Disabilities Research & Practice, 13,* 204–219.

82. Vaughn, S., & Fuchs, L.S. (2003). Redefining learning disabilities as inadequate response to instruction: The promise and potential problems. Learning Disabilities Research & Practice, 18(3), 137–146.
83. Fuchs, D., Fuchs, L.S., & Vaughn, S. (Eds). (2008). Response to intervention: *A framework for reading educators.* (p. 1). Newark, DE. International Reading Association.
84. Lichtenstein, R., & Klotz, M.B. (November 2007). Deciphering the federal regulations on identifying children with specific learning disabilities. NASP Communiqué, Vol. 36, #3.
85. Fletcher, J.M. & Vaugh, S. (2009). Response to intervention models as alternatives to traditional views of learning disabilities: responses to the commentaries. *Child Development Perspectives,* Vol 3, Number 1, pp. 48–50.
86. Barth, A.E., Stuebing, K.K., Anthony, J.L., Denton, C.A., Mathes, P.G., Fletcher, J.M., & Francis, D.J. (2008). Agreement among response to intervention criteria for identifying responder status. *Learning and Individual Differences, 18,* 296–307.
87. Hughes, C. and Dexter, D.D. (2014). The use of RTI to identify students with learning disabilities: a review of the research. *rtinetwork.org.* Retrieved from http://rtinetwork.org/learn/research/use-rti-identify-students-learning-disabilities-review-research.
88. Fuchs, D., & Deshler, D.D. (2007). What we need to know about responsiveness to intervention (and shouldn't be afraid to ask). *Learning Disabilities Research & Practice, 22,* 129–136.
89. Hughes, C. & Dexter, D.D. (2014) The use of RTI to identify students with learning disabilities: a review of the research. http://rtinetwork.org/learn/research/use-rti-identify-students-learning-disabilities-review-research.
90. Hughes, C. and Dexter, D.D. (2014).
91. Ross, A.D. (1976). *Psychological aspects of learning disabilities and reading disorders.* New York: McGraw-Hill.
92. Ysseldyke, J.E., Thurlow, M., Graden, J., Wesson, C., Algozzine, B., & Deno, S. L. (1983). Generalizations from five years of research on assessment and decision making: The University of Minnesota Institute. *Exceptional Education Quarterly, 4(1),* 75–93, p. 89.
93. Lovitt, T. C. (1978). Reactions to planned research. Minneapolis: Institute for Research on Learning Disabilities. Paper presented at the Roundtable Conference on Learning Disabilities. (p.3).
94. Kirk, S.A. (1963). See also: http://spe550.wikispaces.com/file/view/samuel+kirk+article+specific+learning+disaiblities.pdf. See also: Kirk, S.A. Specific learning disabilities. *Journal of Clinical Child Psychology,* Winter 1977, p. 23.

95. Kirk's full statement reads as follows: "Recently, I have used the term 'learning disability' to describe a group of children who have disorders in developmental language, speech, reading and associated communication skills needed for social interaction. In this group I do not include children who have sensory handicaps such as blindness or deafness. ... I also exclude from this group children who have generalized mental retardation" (Kirk, 1963, pp. 2–3).

96. Kirk, S.A. (1963). Behavioral diagnosis and remediation of learning disabilities. *Proceedings of the Conference on Exploration into Problems of the Perceptually Handicapped.* Chicago, IL: Fund for the Perceptually Handicapped.

97. Introduction to learning disabilities. (2006/2007)... *nasetorg.* Retrieved from http://www.naset.org/2522.0.html.

98. Kirk, S. A. & Gallagher, J. J. (1989). Educating exceptional children. Boston: Houghton Mifflin Company, p. 184.

99. Introduction to learning disabilities. (2006/2007)... *nasetorg.* Retrieved from http://www.naset.org/2522.0.html.

100. Various test can confirm or refute the presence of a bacterial infection. Arterial blood test, complete blood count (CBC), blood and sputum cultures, CT scans, among other measures.

101. Retrieved from http://www.naset.org/2522.0.html.

102. Bender, L. (1957). Specific reading disability as a maturational lag. *Bulletin of the Orton Society, 7*, 9–18.

103. Orton, S.T. (1937) *Reading, writing, and speech problems in children.* New York: W.W. Norton.

104. Delcato, C.H. (1959) *The treatment and prevention of reading problems.* Springfield, IL: Charles C Thomas.

105. Schrag, P. and Divoky, D. (1975). p. 39.

106. Ballas, Paul (April 2, 2008). "ADHD's Dynamic History: The Effects of Continuously Changing Diagnostic Criteria". *Health Central.* Remedy Health Media.

107. Barkley, R.A. (2006). Attention Deficit Hyperactivity Disorder: A Handbook for Diagnosis and Treatment (3rd ed.). New York: Guilford Press. See also: http://en.wikipedia.org/wiki/History_of_attention_deficit_hyperactivity_disorder.

108. Lange, Klaus W; Reichl, Susanne; Lange, Katharina M; Tucha, Lara; Tucha, Oliver (November 30, 2010). "The history of attention deficit hyperactivity disorder". *Attention Deficit Hyperactivity Disorders 2* (4): 241–55.

109. Iannelli, V. (2017). A history and medication timeline of ADHD. *verywell.com* Retrieved from https://www.verywell.com/adhd-history-of-adhd-2633127.

110. Alcantara, J. (2008) Attention deficit hyperactivity disorder. *icpa4kids.org* Retrieved from http://icpa4kids.org/Wellness-Articles/attention-deficit-hyperactivity-disorder.html.

111. Sleeter, C.E. (1986). Learning disabilities: The social construction of a special education category. *Exceptional Children, 53,* 46–64.

112. Parker, W. (November 6, 2016). Dyslexia News & Updates: Parents Call for Support on Dyslexic Students. *Parent Herald.* Retrieved from http://www.parentherald.com/articles/81613/20161106/parents-call-support-dyslexic-students.htm.

113. Medical definition of dyslexia. (2016). *medicinenet.org.* Retrieved from http://www.medicinenet.com/script/main/art.asp?articlekey=3138.

114. Causes of dyslexia. (2016). *Dyslexia-reading-well.org.* Retrieved from http://www.dyslexia-reading-well.com/causes-of-dyslexia.html.

115. Knapton, S. (posted February 10, 2015). Dyslexia may not exist. *The Telegraph.* See: http://www.telegraph.co.uk/education/educationnews/10661412/Dyslexia-may-not-exist-warn-academics.html.

116. Personal communication from Daniel Hallahan. (11/11/16) "I suggest that the field should focus on preserving and, in fact, enhancing core principles of special education. I further suggest that those core principles be intensive, individualized instruction. Both of these have been at the heart of special education throughout its history. But both have eroded over the past several decades."

117. Hallahan, D.H. & Mercer, C.D. (2001).

118. Heward, W.L. (July 20, 2010).

119. Hallahan, D.P. & Mercer, C.D. (2001).

120. Doris, J.L. (1993). Defining learning disabilities: A history of the search for consensus. In G.R. Lyon, D.B. Gray, J.F. Kavanagh, & N.A. Krasnegor (Eds.), *Better understanding learning disabilities: New views from research and their implications for education and public policies.* (pp. 97–115). Baltimore, MD: Paul H. Brooks.

121. Mather, N., & Roberts, R. (1994). Learning disabilities: A field in danger of extinction. *Learning Disabilities Research & Practice, 9,* 49–58.

122. Author/date unknown. Attributed to Learning Disability Association of America.

CHAPTER 4

ADHD

The noted seventeenth-century intellectual, Francis Bacon, once suggested that

> "[t]he human understanding when it has once adopted an opinion ... draws all things else to support and agree with it. And though there be a greater number and weight of instances to be found on the other side, yet these it either neglects and despises, or else by some distinction sets aside and rejects."[1]

With that instructive thought in mind, we turn to ADHD and the question of its authenticity, a provocative query in many circles. Most discussions involving the perplexing acronym are more often emotional than learned, leaving them at their heated end precisely where they were at their heated beginning. Testimony, it seems, either to ADHD's uncertainties, or our obstinate biases. Whichever it is, the rancor speaks for itself (Box 4.1).

Box 4.1 ADHD

Pro	Con
People say that ADHD can't be real ... because there's no [biological marker] for it. That's tremendously naïve and it shows a great deal of illiteracy about science.[2]	[The proposal that] ADHD is a biological or neurological disorder is entirely fabricated.[3] Psychiatrist Peter Breggin suggests ADHD is more a social construct than it is an objective "disorder."[4,5]

Box 4.1   (continued)

Pro	Con
"As a matter of science, the notion that ADHD does not exist is simply wrong."[6]	Dr. Leon Eisenberg, the "father" of ADHD, stated that ADHD "is a prime example of a fictitious disease."[7]
To suggest that [ADHD] is a fraud, that somehow children are being abused by these treatments, is really an outrage, because for these kids, to not get treated is really the greatest abuse and neglect.[8]	If ever any country badly needs a sobering dose of science about ADHD to temper overenthusiastic diagnosis and treatment, it is the United States. Those of us who helped start [the ADHD boom] look at their out-of-control American progeny with something akin to the horror of the creator of Frankenstein.[9]
"Claims that ADHD is not a valid disorder are egregiously wrong and … show either a stunning scientific illiteracy or a planned religious or political propaganda intended to deceive the uninformed or unsuspecting public."[10]	Despite repeated reports in the press that a neurological cause for ADHD has been identified,[11] there is no persuasive evidence that children diagnosed with ADHD differ from other children in any identifiable neurological or biochemical manner.[12]
ADHD has been described by notable professionals as a "genuine" condition[13] that is both "true"[14] and "real."[15]	*ADHD Does Not Exist.*[16]
Attention-deficit/hyperactivity disorder (ADHD) is a real disease linked to changes in production of the brain chemical dopamine, two new reports suggest.[17]	The Australian National Association of Practising Psychiatrists (NAPP): "[ADHD] is not an inherited genetic disorder or organic disease" and "scientific evidence to support ADHD as a disorder is unproven."[18]
"Attention deficit hyperactivity is real. Don't let anyone tell you otherwise."[19]	Psychiatrist Denis Donovan, MD: "ADD is a bogus diagnosis. Parents and teachers are rushing like lemmings to identify a pathology. … Our current pathologizing of behavior leads to massive swelling of the ranks of the diseased, the dysfunctional, the disordered and the disabled."[20]

(continued)

Box 4.1 (continued)

Pro	Con
Though often ridiculed, ADHD represents a genuine medical condition that robs people of major life chances.[21]	"The past 25 years has led to a phenomenon almost unique in history. Methodologically rigorous research … indicates that ADD [attention-deficit disorder] and hyperactivity as 'syndromes' simply do not exist. We have invented a disease, given it medical sanction, and now must disown it. The major question is how we go about destroying the monster we have created. It is not easy to do this and still save face."[22]
[Referencing Dr. Peter Breggin, MD, Psychiatrist, "ADHD is a misdiagnosis," *NY Times*, October 13, 2011. COMMENTS]. "Do you have it Dr. Breggin? How do you dare to tell me I don't? Who are you to tell me I haven't suffered because of ADHD? You know nothing about my pain. Don't tell me about the pain I didn't have, as I failed night and day with this thing you swear doesn't exist. You have no idea, my friend. None."[23]	"I'm reluctant to write a post about ADHD. It … seems like treacherous ground. … Expressing an opinion about this diagnosis … will be met with criticism from one side or another. If … we don't make a diagnosis of ADHD, but instead document that the child has 'problems in focusing' or 'inattention' or 'hyperactivity,' then it behooves us to continue looking for the causes of those symptoms. For some children, it may be a chaotic home environment. For others, it may be a history of neglect, or ongoing substance abuse. For others, it may be a parenting style or interaction which is not ideal for that child's social or biological makeup. (I hesitate to write 'poor parenting' because then I'll *really* get hate mail!)"[24] (Steve Balt, MD, Psychiatrist)

- ADHD has been called a malady, a disease, a syndrome, a disorder, a medical condition. It's been called a fiction. It's been called a social construct. It's been called an excuse. It's been called a hoax.
- Eighty-five scientists from leading universities in 13 countries recognized the mounting evidence of neurological and genetic contributions to ADHD. … To publish stories that ADHD is a fictitious disorder … is tantamount to declaring the earth flat, the laws of gravity debatable, and the periodic table in chemistry a fraud.[25]

- ADHD is said to be caused by a malfunctioning brain, irregular genes, inadequate sleep, weed killer found in food supply, low birthrate (under 5.5 lbs), maternal drinking, smoking during pregnancy, second-hand smoke, iron deficiencies, lead in bloodstream, protein malnutrition, sleep deficiencies, and dyes. Sugar (apparently) is *not* a cause.[26] Pesticides, flame-retardant chemicals, and insecure bonds early in life have been proposed as causes. Likewise, fluorescent lights, television, chemical cleaners, antibiotics, heavy metals, depleted vitamins, minerals, and fatty acids, and not enough time in the great outdoors. Not surprisingly, chiropractors have argued that "spinal misalignment" and a "misaligned skull" are responsible for ADHD.[27]

  (FYI: "Chiropractic therapy isn't likely to harm your child. However, there is no clear evidence to show that it can help kids with learning and attention issues.")[28]

  Other prognosticators have pointed to prolonged birth labor, umbilical cord issue, meningitis, head injury, low parental education level, poverty, parenting styles, and a "rapid-fire culture."[29]
- ADHD is said to be overdiagnosed.[30] ADHD is said to be underdiagnosed.[31] ADHD is said to be overmedicated.[32] ADHD is said to be undermedicated.[33]
- It's been said that ADHD's diagnostic procedures reflect good science. It's been said that the various elements that comprise the syndrome—inefficiency at school—are seldom, if ever, observed directly, let alone measured, by the diagnosing physician. It's been said that the [diagnostic] criteria are … by their very nature, subjective.[34] It's been said that worrisome, authentic diagnostic procedures are weakened by hurried, subjective opinions evoked under intense pressure brought to bear by parents and/or teachers who demand immediate answers and resolution.[35,36]
- It's been said that "[preschoolers] offer a real opportunity for early [ADHD] identification and treatment to prevent years of academic failure. It's been said that preschoolers are ripe for overdiagnosis and overmedication."[37]
- It's been said that ADHD affects children as young as 2.[38] It's been said that ADHD is neonatal; it's been said that it is fetal.[39] Officially, 36 months is its entry point, safe to treat with medication, so it's been said.[40,41] More than 10,000 American toddlers 2 or 3 years old are being medicated for ADHD outside established pediatric guidelines, according to data presented by the Center for Disease Control and Prevention.[42]

- It's been said that drugs are safe; it's been said drugs are not safe.[43,44,45] It's been said that the long-term effects are largely unknown.[46] "Safer than aspirin," a psychiatrist once said when speaking of the drug Adderall. He later remarked, "I regret the analogy and won't be saying that again."[47]
- It's been said that America today suffers from culturally induced attention-deficit disorder, or what [is] called "pseudo-ADD."[48]
- It's been said that those who truly suffer from this condition stand to lose tremendously if the public ... trivializes the disorder ... [and] comes to see ADHD as nothing more than a label applied to an individual who experiences frustration with himself or herself or with his or her children.[49]
- It's been said that ADHD is not a disease like diabetes. It's been said that ADHD represents behaviors that create a poor fit between the child and his or her parents and teachers, and which often annoy and frustrate adults. Sometimes, these behaviors are normal variants in temperament, sometimes they are behavior skills that have not been sufficiently trained and sometimes there are underlying learning, emotional, medical or relational problems which manifest in ADHD-like symptoms. Whichever the explanation, it is almost never the case that there is something fundamentally wrong with the child. The good news is that whatever the underlying [reason], parents can truly become the primary agents of change in the child's life![50]
- It's been said that ADHD, used as a primary diagnosis, has no etiologic significance, is conceptually and diagnostically distracting, leads to a paucity of thinking about a patient's early developmental history and trauma, and is therapeutically misleading.[51]
- It's been said to be a ministering angel: "Being diagnosed with ADD gave me my life back. ... At last my problem has a name and it's not my fault."[52]

***

Recently, renowned Harvard psychologist Jerome Kagan, mincing no words, said that ADHD is largely a fraud. He believes that the most modern diagnosis is a mere invention rather than a serious condition, an invention that mainly benefits the pharmaceutical industry and psychiatrists. "Every child who's not doing well in school is sent to a pediatrician who says, 'It's ADHD; here's Ritalin'." Dr. Kagan added that 90% of these 5.4 million* kids don't have an abnormal dopamine metabolism. The problem is that if a drug is available to doctors, they'll make the corresponding diagnosis.[53] (*Federal statistics estimate that some 6.4 million American children, aged 3–17, have been diagnosed with ADHD.[54])

In support of Dr. Kagan, physician Michael Anderson calls the disorder (ADHD) "made up" and "an excuse" to prescribe the pills to treat what he considers the children's true ill—poor academic performance in inadequate schools. Dr. Anderson said that every child he treats with ADHD medication has met qualifications. But he also railed against those criteria, saying they were codified only to "make something completely subjective look objective."[55]

Child neurologist Fred Baughman estimates thus: "We've got probably, conservatively … six million [children in the United States] on medications for ADHD, and a total of nine million with neurobiologic psychiatric diagnoses of one sort or another on one or more psychotropic drugs. Here we're talking about as many kids as you've got people in New York City. And to me, this is a catastrophe. These are all normal children."[56]

Harvard professor and psychiatrist Robert Berezin has suggested,

> Somewhere along the line we have lost the understanding that kids come in all shapes and sizes. Some kids are active, some are quiet; some kids are dreamers, others are daring; some kids are dramatic, others are observers; some impulsive, others reserved; some leaders, others followers; some athletic, others thinkers. Where did we ever get the notion that kids should all be one way?
>
> "Poor parents these days are subject to pediatric 'experts' who proclaim that kids should follow some prescribed rates of physical, mental, and emotional growth. If they deviate from the 'mean,' then there is a problem. Parents are intimidated and worry that there is something wrong with their babies. Every child matures in his own way, in his own time. Every child is different. We need to throw away all the bell curves of 'normal.' There is no such thing as ADHD."[57]

Offering a contrary perspective, psychiatrist Peter Jensen suggests: "Diseases of the mind [ADHD] shouldn't be treated any differently than the diseases of the other parts of the body."[58] His medical view is supported by child psychologist Steven Kurtz, Senior Director of the ADHD and Disruptive Behavior Disorders Center at the Child Mind Institute, who suggests: "We need to see ADHD as a condition like high blood pressure, or high cholesterol or diabetes."[59]

Adding to the confusion, we've been informed that a variety of other disorders can masquerade as ADHD.[60] Most troubling is the assertion that a child's behaviors may be mistaken for ADHD when, in fact, they're a cry for help.

Dr. Nancy Rappaport, a child psychiatrist and director of school-based programs at Cambridge Health Alliance outside Boston who specializes in underprivileged youth, said that some home environments can lead to behavior often mistaken for ADHD, particularly in the youngest children:

> In acting out and being hard to control, [the children are] signaling the chaos in their environment. ... [I]f you have a family with domestic violence, drug or alcohol abuse, or a parent neglecting a 2-year-old, the kid might look impulsive or aggressive. And the parent might just want a quick fix, and the easiest thing to do is medicate. It's a travesty.[61]

As if these conflicting perspectives weren't enough to make your head cartwheel, we're told that politics, prejudice, ignorance, and dollars influence whether a child said to be ADHD receives any services, a situation we'd rarely expect to happen with typical childhood illnesses.

In 2014, medical writer Brenda Goodman reported that "[c]hildren without health insurance were less likely to be diagnosed with ADHD than children who had coverage. Kids from lower-income families were also less likely to be diagnosed. ... Children with older mothers, who tend to be more highly educated, and those with parents who spoke to doctors in English were more likely to be diagnosed with [ADHD]. White kids were [much more likely] to be diagnosed than Asian, Hispanic or Black kids." I asked myself what there was about a family's income, its prime language, its maternal member's education, its culture, and its health insurance that had to do with saying a child within the family had or didn't have ADHD? If the ailment was measles, would medical doctors be blind to all factors outside the infection? Are Asian, Hispanic, or Black parents less likely to accept (or buy into) the notion of disorder? Or is the disparity related to ADHD's well-documented subjective diagnostic methodology? A study published in April 2012 in the *Canadian Medical Association Journal* found that the youngest children in their school class were more likely to be diagnosed [ADHD] compared to the oldest children in those grades, suggesting that some doctors and teachers may mistake immaturity for ADHD, leading to overdiagnosis, Ms. Goodman added.[62]

* * *

For many of us, this quarreling over ADHD's credibility is both surprising and unsettling. We're not accustomed to professionals bickering over what should be a straightforward answer to a pressing concern, especially one that involves a child and his/her stressful behavior. Our experiences with our own children prompt us to predict the opposite. If our child presents a physical complaint, we anticipate a ready solution without any accompanying controversy. We take our youngster to see the family physician. Within minutes (or a day or two) we're told, "Katie has this." Thankfully, we most often hear, "Not to worry. This is what we'll do about it," the certainty of the answer most comforting. We expect nothing less. As a result of these generally positive outcomes, we've been lulled into the belief that we could present to a handful of expertly trained professionals the same concerns about a child, provide the experts the same answers to their same questions, and receive mostly the same replies from each. When second opinions confirm first opinions, we're buoyed with confidence.

Unfortunately, we're not likely to experience this relished professional consistency when the topic of ADHD is broached. Troubling as this sounds, we could interview two physicians, discuss the same questions and concerns about a child, and receive contrary explanations, along with contrary suggestions regarding treatment. Visiting with two psychologists, we could experience equally divergent answers. Two special education teachers, the same. Books, articles, opinions, editorials, the same confusing, contradictory conclusions and advice. You might ask "How is it possible that professionals hold such varying opinions?" It does seem curious. After all, we're not talking about a rare tropical disease that affects a tiny population in a faraway land. Most assuredly, the contrary is the case.

- We're talking about many millions of American children with an ADHD diagnosis.
- We're talking about a presumed condition with a purported biogenetic base that some experts suggest warrants pharmaceutical intervention as the front-line treatment—even with 2-year-olds.

Those who are bothered by all this discordant noise can't help but wonder, "What is this ADHD?" My answer: "Don't expect a simple answer."

ADHD: The Name

We've become obsessed with what ADHD means. Don't we first have to figure out what it is?[63]

I believe efforts to introduce ADD (ADHD) to the public have opened a Pandora's box. In attempting to package for public consumption a condition that psychiatry is still struggling to define—and for which it has a long list of symptoms but no firm explanation—the popularizers have contributed to widespread confusion about just what ADD/(ADHD) is and who can be said to "have" it.[64]

The late American psychiatrist Thomas Szasz noted: "The suggestion that ... [ADHD] is not a disease at all—is politically so incorrect that it is dismissed out of hand."[65]

Dr John Jureidini, head of the Department of Psychological Medicine at the Women's and Children's Hospital, Adelaide, South Australia, responding to a question raised by a parliamentary commission:
"There is monumental literature that takes as a given that ADHD is a neurobiological condition and starts from there to talk about different forms of treatment. Once you have many thousands of articles published about something, how can it possibly make sense for someone to stand up and say, 'This is not an entity'? I want to emphasise that I quite clearly acknowledge that there are children who are very compromised because of difficulties with impulsiveness, attention and activity. I am not saying that these children are not suffering or are not worthy of attention. I am saying that, as a disorder, ADHD is a spurious entity."[66]

ADHD, in a fundamental sense, is a name, more correctly, an assigned acronym representing "attention-deficit hyperactive disorder." Some clinicians prefer simply ADD where hyperactivity is not a current characteristic of a school child. Rather than discovered and biologically validated in a medical laboratory as are most named physiological disorders, ADHD, the acronym, was voted on and christened at a meeting of the American Psychiatric Association in 1980. The policy that results in such names and acronyms goes this way. A group of psychiatrists get together every few years at their national convention and sit down in a room and decide what behaviors they think should be considered psychiatric disorders. This group of psychiatrists votes to include certain groups of behaviors as psychiatric disorders and make up names for these disorders.[67] You should know that these meetings have had a quarrelsome history, perhaps foretelling ADHD's current lack of professional agreement.

The professionals who create, name and/or revise these diagnostic categories are recruited by the American Psychiatric Association. Political considerations, as well as professional relationships and rivalries, inevitably enter the selection process. Factions that disagree on a disorder's legitimacy may sit on the same committee, and decisions are sometimes made for reasons other than strict science. Efforts at being diagnostically objective have been quite subjective.[68]

The particular acronym, ADHD, has been revised on two separate occasions since its inception, in 1987 and 1994.[69] That it has been amended twice to date offers evidence of measured disagreement among the small group of medically trained voters, the object of their dispute related to what ADHD ought to be and what it ought not to be, easy grounds for friction where one's professional turf and scientific principles are challenged.

Understand, please, that the lack of professional accord does *not* lie with the acronym. "ADHD" was psychiatry's choice, initially used by the field as a convenience, an umbrella term, similar in kind to what Sam Kirk had in mind for his "learning disability." Most any acronym chosen by psychiatry would have sufficed. Its only prerequisite that it represents whatever the naming-committee thought was relative and important. These acronyms do serve a valuable purpose. Notice the following.

(FYI: The medical acronym "PANDAS" is by far more conversationally friendly than what the acronym represents: "Pediatric, Autoimmune Neuropsychiatric Disorder Associated with Streptococcal Infection.")

As such, ADHD (attention-deficit hyperactivity disorder), CP (cerebral palsy), LD (learning disability), and PANDAS, are shorthand representational terms that make conversation easier. Though helpful in that respect, please understand that "ADHD," like CP and LD, is not a very useful descriptive term, not if we wish to understand more thoroughly the child we're talking about. Similar to what was mention in the previous chapter, gather ten "ADHD-kids" around the park's flagpole, and you'll have ten mostly different kids, their behavioral and attentional topographies often very dissimilar. What is noticeable about ADHD, again not unlike LD, laypeople and professionals alike hold discernibly diverse opinions as to what constitutes ADHD, that is, which behavioral and attentional variations best fit with the acronym. The lack of behavioral (symptom) consistency has been noted.

> Critics of the diagnosis have argued that ADHD diagnostic criteria [are] sufficiently general or vague to allow virtually anybody with persistent unwanted behaviors to be classified as having ADHD of one type or another.[70]

Since ADHD can be pretty much what anyone wants it to be, its eventual status is for others to argue—and others, as you've seen, will argue, with contrary sides represented:

- Psychologist Terrie Moffitt, along with epidemiologist Maria Melchior, declared that ADHD is "a bona fide mental disorder (as opposed to a social construction)."[71]
- Conversely, psychologist Dathan Paterno,[72] along with physician Olavo Amaral when writing in the *American Journal of Psychiatry*,[73] declared the contrary, that ADHD *is* a social construct and not a disorder, differences, again, that we've come to expect.

(FYI: Recall that social constructs are terms that represent complex topics such as race, culture, love, cancer, aggression, compassion, autism, sex, peace, drugs and rock and roll. Most important, constructs are *never* directly observed, and are defined entirely by whatever their user had in mind. Perhaps that explains why "politics" and "religion" are often unvited guests to a fun social party.)

It's your choice to enter into or abstain from the debate that argues whether ADHD is a real biological disorder or a complex social construct that was conceived by 20th century psychiatry. If you're uncertain, I'll make this first part easy for you, allowing the definition, *not* my bias, to be the tiebreaker.

As you've read, ADHD is a generated name, or more precisely an acronym, psychiatry's choice. It's an acronym that replaced an earlier generated name that itself replaced an even earlier generated name. In that sense, ADHD is a chameleon-like social construct that psychiatry adjusts whenever it chooses to do so. One might predict another modification will come along within the next few years. According to scientific principles, therefore, ADHD, in its present form, is not an established, measurable biological entity, and therefore not a bona fide disorder that's been verified in a medical laboratory. (If you wish to argue that point, please read David Mechanic's piece further on in this chapter. His perspective might be helpful.)

ADHD is what it was intended to be, a representational term, like PANDAS. You and others must decide what the term represents, perhaps a child's disobedient actions, or his nasty temperament, or her unkindly attitude, or all three, along with a dozen other features.

Attention deficit with hyperactivity suggests a common, broad syndrome, but in fact this cannot be sustained as a biological entity. [It] is not coherent in its symptomatology; it is not reliably diagnosed in practice; it has not been shown to have predictive value separately from the ... conduct problems which frequently coexist; and its associations are with psychosocial adversity as much as with biological disadvantage.[74]

While much about ADHD is arguable, this much is not: it is ubiquitous and as Malcolm Gladwell suggested, we are obsessed with it. Though conceding that it's widespread, those of us who like our stereotypical "I"'s dotted" and our "T's crossed" are left uncomfortably confused by this acronym that has created such heated debates. Without much "skin" in the game beyond the acronym's authenticity, we'd like some reasonable evidence that would verify this created acronym's structure. We'd like to point to it and say, "Hey, there it is." Not yet, I must share. Despite everyone's best efforts to place ADHD's illustrative profile within a picture frame, this term psychiatry coined years ago remains elusive. Psychiatrist Edward M. Hallowell suggested that those whose job it is to pin down ADHD are more like—

> blind men describing an elephant. The elephant is there—this ... collection of people with varying attentional strengths and vulnerabilities. However, generating a definitive description, diagnostic workup, and treatment plan ... pose a challenge.[75]

Be that as it may, ADHD has been embraced with extraordinary zealousness by professionals and laypeople alike, often with little consistency. With its many faces, found in so many places, psychiatrist Hallowell suggested:

> The diagnosis has become so seductive that it sometimes seems more like a designer label on a piece of clothing than a real, potentially disabling disorder.[76]

Be the sartorial reference true or otherwise, one troubling fact cannot be denied: many of our children are in the crosshairs. There's one overriding concern that is often lost when our ADHD acrimonious debates rage, where making our point becomes the sole object of our energies. Regardless of the circumstances that call forth the acronym, invariably, there's a child whose displayed behaviors are taxing to a parent, a teacher, or both. Stating the obvious early, ADHD, in whatever form it takes, *never* finds itself in the company of a child whose exemplary behaviors meet or exceed a parent's or teacher's personal standard. That this standard is unique to the individual teacher or parent translates to a wildly elastic barometer, assuring ADHD's persona a wide latitude. That's not in anyone's interest. What a physician or psychologist interprets as ADHD-like behavior, a parent sees otherwise. What a parent reports as ADHD, the two professionals fail to see.

Interestingly, we don't have that same problem with, say, croup or ear infections or a dislocated thumb. Why that's the case warrants some thought. Part of the answer may be that croup, ear infections, and the awkward thumb have built-in markers and boundaries that keep each in its respective place. A dislocated thumb is a dislocated thumb, and it's rarely interpreted as anything else. Conversely, ADHD, without similarly apparent boundaries and markers, seems to find itself everywhere, even in places where it's either uninvited or where it should be uninvited. Consider today's ADHD in the USA. There's much about it that's worrisome.

A mother received a phone call from the principal at her son's preschool to report that her three-year-old was "acting up" and "disrupting class." The principal wanted the parents to come in for a meeting because she suspected that the child *had* ADHD. "He really stuck out like a sore thumb," the principal said. "Your son's approach is to bombard everyone with his presence." The boy's father is from France where children are rarely diagnosed with mental disorders. It didn't occur to him that there was anything wrong with his son. "He's just a boy and he's very active and ... we didn't think much of it," the father said. After discussing their son's situation with the school, the family met with a psychologist—an ADHD specialist. At first, the psychologist thought the child might be attending the wrong school. But after he saw a videotape of the boy in the classroom, he said: "It was pretty apparent that he was below average in his ability to just stay in one place." In order to determine if the boy *had* ADHD, the psychologist proposed using a standard diagnostic tool—the Conners Rating Scale, a checklist of 28 behaviors like "restless in the squirmy sense," "overly sensitive to criticism," "childish and immature." "The psychologist suggested he might be ADD or ADHD, which were new acronyms for us," the mother reported. "And then he suggested the use of medication. For us, it was like a cold shower," said the mother. The boy's parents chose not to formally test him for ADHD. "He's a handful," said the boy's father. "He is more intense. He is more active. ... But I could never understand how that would translate into my son having something wrong with his brain."[77]

***

On a family's kitchen shelf, next to the peanut butter and chicken broth, sits a wire basket brimming with bottles of the children's medications: Adderall for a daughter, 12, and her brother, who's 9; Risperdal (an antipsychotic for mood stabilization) for twin 11-year-old boys; and Clonidine (a sleep aid to counteract other medications) prescribed for all four children, taken nightly. One of the twins ("Buddy") began taking Adderall for ADHD when he was 6, when his disruptive school behavior led to calls home and in-school suspensions. He immediately settled down and became a more earnest, attentive student—a little bit more like his twin brother, who also took Adderall for his ADHD. When puberty's chemical maelstrom began at about 10 years of age, Buddy got into fights at school because, he said, other children were insulting his mother. Investigated, the problem was they were *not* insulting the boy's mother. Buddy was seeing people and hearing voices that were not there, a rare but recognized side effect of Adderall. After Buddy admitted to being suicidal, the prescribing physician admitted the child to a local psychiatric hospital for a week and switched the boy to Risperdal. While telling this story, the parents called Buddy into the kitchen and asked him to describe why he had been given Adderall.

"To help me focus on my school work, my homework, listening to Mom and Dad, and not doing what I used to do to my teachers, to make them mad," he said. "If I don't take my medicine I'd be having attitudes. I'd be disrespecting my parents. I wouldn't be like this." Despite Buddy's [experiences] with Adderall, the family decided to use it with their 12-year-old daughter and 9-year-old son.

These children don't have ADHD, their parents said. The Adderall is merely to help their grades, and because the daughter was, in her father's words, "a little blah."

"We've seen both sides of the spectrum: We've seen positive, we've seen negative," the father said. Acknowledging that his daughter's use of Adderall is "cosmetic," he added, "[i]f they're feeling positive, happy, socializing more, and it's helping them, why wouldn't you? Why not?"[78]

- I am 25, and my 4-year old son and I have ADHD, we are both on amphetamines. I love it, my son is the little boy I knew I always had but was never able to "see." ... This has helped my little man ... not have outbursts and break things anymore.
- I have four kids who are all ADHD. I love this drug [Ritalin].
- Mom-1: It is normal for toddlers to seem as if they are ADD/ADHD. They will not usually medicate a child until they have reached age 5 or 6.

  Mom-2: Don't pay attention to the jerk above. ... My son started on his meds around 3.

  Mom-3: A psychiatrist diagnosed my son with ADHD when he was 2 and a half. ... He has been medicated for 3 years now and it does wonders.

- "It's scary to think that this is what we've come to; how not funding public education to meet the needs of all kids has led to this," said the superintendent of one major school district in California who spoke on the condition of anonymity. Referring to the use of stimulants in children without classic ADHD, the superintendent said: "I don't know, but it could be happening right here. Maybe not as knowingly, but it could be a consequence of a doctor who sees a kid failing in overcrowded classes with 42 other kids and the frustrated parents asking what they can do. The doctor says, 'Maybe it's A.D.H.D., let's give this a try.'"[79] The doctor says it's worth a try; that carries a lot of influence. But there's the negative side to the use of that which helps to improve a child's performance—the still unknown long-term effects on developing brain tissue, according to the American Academy of Pediatrics.[80]

OMAHA, NEBRASKA

It's not often that one stands at a transformation's dawn: The Wright brothers' initial winged box that defied gravity; the first human squawk that traversed Alexander Graham Bell's raw wire. In retrospect, though admittedly personalized, what my fellow graduate students and I witnessed felt nearly as dramatic. We caught the first ripple of the tsunami, the wave that was to come, the wave that has come. It was the late 60s. Initially, the announcement was an amusement, mostly a curiosity. We, of course, weren't privy to the future, what would eventually affect the lives of so many children and parents around the world.

A mounted bulletin board in Arizona State University's Educational Psychology office kept graduate students abreast of important happenings. We read postings that included guest speakers on campus, dates and locations of upcoming local and professional meetings, announcements related to exam schedules, grants awarded, lab partners sought, PhD defenses, and an occasional humorous item related to the field. I don't recall whether the brief notice found itself in the humor section or whether a professor with prescient powers provided the news blurb to alert us:

"TAKE NOTICE—IMPORTANT"

The article in the newspaper read (something close to):

Nebraskan pediatrician uses amphetamines to help a young schoolboy do better in school, dubbing the medication: "The thinking drug."

We were puzzled. What was there to medicate? We knew amphetamines. The small band of us attached to the behavior laboratory certainly knew how to improve a child's school behavior. It didn't require drugs. Despite our youthful incredulity, whatever was happening in Cornhusker-land established itself as does a sapling, its foundation deep enough for the tap-root to worm its way to Washington, D.C. Two years later, in 1970 precisely (most of us having taken positions in university departments across the U.S.), the *Washington Post* published a story describing how 5–10% of *all* school children in Omaha, Nebraska, were receiving the stimulant medication Ritalin to "control their behavior" in the classroom. Ratcheting the hysteria, the newspaper article insinuated that many parents were being coerced into medicating their kids.[81] The resulting outrage was enough to produce a federal inquiry.[82] The federal government, however, suffers its own attention-deficit; their interest fizzled like a damp firecracker.

The published findings streaming out of Omaha had far-reaching implications. Medical and educational authorities around the country reported that they, too, noticed that some kids taking low dose stimulants did do better in school, their behavior improved, as did their studies, the outcome embraced by teachers exhausted from undisciplined children. The observation prompted medical model professionals to conclude:

- The children's brains were wired differently.
- The children were biologically disabled.
- A diagnostic tool had been discovered to support the hypothesis that the children suffered "minimal brain damage."

The debate involving ADHD, the acronym still several years away, had begun to heat up.

Summary We've more than followed the Nebraska pediatrician's innovative, if not controversial, lead. Stimulant medication is widely used by today's schoolchildren, some designated ADHD, and many others where ADHD isn't stipulated or considered.

The sales of ADHD prescription medication are increasing rapidly and are expected to grow by another 13 percent this year alone. According to *IBIS World*, a new report shows ADHD medication has skyrocketed since 2010, and will continue to grow at an annualized rate of 6 percent per year, bringing in $17.5 billion by the year 2020.[83]

Data from the federal Center for Disease Control (CDC) has suggested that approximately 6% of 2011 school children take stimulant medication, presumably to either modify their behavior or promote school performance. Current reported figures (2013–14):

* Kids on psychiatric drugs: **8,389,034**
* **Kids on ADHD drugs: 4,404,360**[84]

The liberal dispensing of the powerful medication, despite its discrete gains, has prompted concerns.

I shudder when I hear my colleagues suggest you can go ahead and give drugs to children to see what their behaviors are like. … We really don't know what are the effects of a lot of these drugs on a lot of processes over the long run.[85] (Charles Hersch, Ph.D., Clinical Psychologist)

HISTORIC ADHD

More than a century before the significant happenings in Nebraska, an event took place in Europe that rooted the medical model into today's classrooms. The published event would be seized upon by American psychiatry and become the prototype from which would spring countless proposed mental and education disabilities that would be used (incorrectly, it must be said) to *explain* a bevy of troublesome school and home-related behaviors. Several early physicians spoke of children with ADHD-like behaviors. British physician George Sills in 1902, for example, thought the unruly behaviors he observed represented "an abnormal defect of moral control in children."[86] And Heinrich Hoffman offered readers (and medical historians) a fictional character he named "Fidgety Phil,"[87] a youngster whose parents needed considerable help dealing with their unruly boy. While other examples were humorous and provocative, one seminal incident proved to be truly historic. It presented the first clear and uncompromising example of the *medicalization* of schoolchildren.[88] If what occurred that day weren't so significant, some of us would advertise the performance as an old-time vaudeville show.

Often touted as the *first* formal example of ADHD,[89,90] the historic moment occurred in the latter part of the eighteenth century in a classroom filled with young children, all dressed in hand-me-down itchy woolen clothing, seated on hardwood chairs or benches, situated in either an overheated room or one cold enough to freeze a side of beef. The compelling story reveals the medical model's shortsightedness, a blurred vision as prevalent today as it was 200 years ago.

Scottish physician, Sir Alexander Crichton (1763–1856), entered a school's classroom where the children were seated as tightly as Norwegian sardines packed in a can. The youngsters' starchy teacher, in black garb that covered every inch of skin from her narrow neck to boney ankles, stood at a tiny chalkboard with a pile of large books on a table that might have accommodated a chessboard.

(FYI: The depiction was taken from an internet picture.)

The rectangular room in the shape of a shoe box forced the strict teacher to turn her back to half her youngsters when she spoke to the opposite sitting children. (Children do notice when their stern teacher is not looking.)

Visiting the classroom, Sir Alex observed several children who *had* what he termed "the fidgets."[91] The teacher, keenly aware of her pupils' antics, pressed the medical man to *explain* why some of her children couldn't keep their small bottoms glued to their seats. Dr. Crichton, a surgeon by training, suffered no loss for words. The angular-faced physician explained to the inquisitive teacher (and all future generations of teachers and physicians) that "*the children's* [frazzled] *state of nerves*"[92] were what caused the youngsters' excessive squirminess and presumed inattention.

In one fell swoop, by way of a singular authoritative declaration issued without constraint, Sir Alexander Crichton laid the foundation for twentieth-century ADHD.[93] He said:

> When born with a person it becomes evident at a very early period of life, and has a very bad effect, in as much as it renders him incapable of attending with constancy to any one object of education.[94]

There it was, the size of a harvest moon served up on an iconic silver platter. A modern-day ADHD advocate, needing historical evidence for his cause, couldn't ask for anything better.

Despite its appeal, that celebrated day does require clarification. Understand that physician Crichton did *not* see the youngsters' frazzled nerves while he watched the children twiddle on their bottoms. He saw precisely what you and I would have seen had we been present in the classroom—how the children behaved during their teacher's lessons. Whereas we can observe what children do, how they behave, in the absence of any independent evidence (e.g., X-rays, blood tests), we must presume the presence of underlying neurological conditions such as the children's "state of nerves." Obviously satisfied to assume the children's nerves caused their inattentiveness, physician Crichton felt no obligation to either question his own conclusions or consider that something else might have contributed to the kids' fidgets. (That's decidedly poor science.) In his defense, the man's medical school professors provided him no options to consider. If you only know biology, you only see biology. (That's a decidedly poor education.)

(FYI: Solid scientists, with no personal agenda, routinely challenge their colleagues to prove their suppositions and research findings *wrong*. If *wrong* can't be empirically produced, despite strenuous efforts and well-controlled studies, the original findings and/or thesis gain credibility. The best example of such was Jonas Salk. Prior to administering to his own wife and children the polio vaccine he had developed, he begged his colleagues to prove his thesis and research findings wrong, understandably since the vaccine he was about to inject into his wife and kids contained the (assumed) "killed" polio virus. Dr. Crichton didn't *man up* to that school of thought. Seeing himself as invulnerable to challenge, he assumed he was right, expecting everyone to agree. A surgeon, yes, but not a man of science.)

We know kids don't twiddle and chatter without reason. Something sets off their disturbing actions. If we had pointed that out to Sir Alex, if we pressed him to think about a possible alternative explanation for the kids' impatient behavior, the medical man might have snapped back, "If not for frazzled nerves, why *else* would the children be so inattentive?" Why else, indeed. Therein lies a major deficiency with the medical model, specifically its failure to consider the possibility that *non*-biological alternatives might have produced the children's restlessness.

(FYI: Alternative explanations for a child's behavior most often lead to alternative strategies. Professionals who provide direct services to kids, who view children's behavior within the *context* of their educational and familial environments, like to have a variety of interventions. If, however, we're what's called a "one-trick pony," how I'd describe Sir Alex, we'd be like the dentist who, without reading the new patients' charts, informs those in the waiting room, "Today's Tuesday. Everyone gets nitrous oxide and root canals." Or in the case of a fidgety or inattentive child, Ritalin.)

CONTEXT

Let me expand on the term "context." It's all-important. Dr. Crichton did *not* observe the snugly grouped children in the isolation of his private medical office, what so often happens with today's physicians, out of necessity, of course. Crichton observed the children in their classroom, an active, if not cramped, space filled with kids and books and papers and assignments, all monitored by their stiff-minded teacher with her own unique style. That's called "context." Context represents the circumstance associated with children's actions, the who, what, when, where, and why of the behavior.

Context, what amounts to everything within an individual's life space, imparts a great influence on what a child does. (It imparts great influence on what you and I do.) Sir Alex, by his own choice, *ignored* context, treating it as an alien world. He figuratively plucked the youngsters from their influential environment, like lifting cubs from their den, thereby judging the children's actions in isolation. He chose to explain their disturbing movements by naming frazzled nerves as the cause of their disruptions, to the exclusion of anything else, a diagnostic assertion that can't be proven wrong or right. (That's also poor science.) Yet, in *his own words*, as you'll now see, Sir Alex undermined his own credibility. He candidly provided an alternative explanation for the children's annoying twiddles, an alternative that any reasonably open-minded professional would have considered long before pronouncing the child neurologically defective, an alternative, by the way, that could be tested to assess its validity. Sir Alex shared, and I'm quoting once again:

> Every public teacher must have observed that there are many [pupils] to whom the dryness and difficulties of the Latin and Greek grammars are so disgusting that neither the terrors of the rod, nor the indulgence of kind intreaty (sic) can cause them to give their attention to them.[95]

Sir Alex's illuminating oration provides at least three options to the children's alleged defective nerves that the medical man claimed prevented the youngsters from giving their teacher or their assignments their undivided attention:

* The children's insufficient curriculum skills.
* The "disgusting" Latin/Greek grammar.
* The children saw no reason to pay attention.

That the physician was blind to the three options reflects his training.

(FYI: Thorough scientists require a minimum of three separate data points before drawing even preliminary conclusions about what they're observing. Did Sir Alex do a controlled series of observations? Did he return to the class two more times to determine if his initial observations were replicated? I found no evidence of that. What would he have concluded if he witnessed all the kids captivated and fixed in place by the teacher's powerpoint presentation? More on that in a moment.)

Though we could test out the merits of the three possible options to Dr. Crichton's flawed nerves, we'll only consider the first two for the time being. Keep in mind that a single exception to an accepted rule creates a crack in that rule, and reason to look further. (That's good science.)

"Q": What might have happened had the starchy teacher provided the kids an exciting, *achievable* curriculum challenge, something to do with the Loch Ness monster or the Royal Scots Regiment or sailing the stormy Firth of Clyde, the purpose to assess if their attentiveness changed even the slightest as compared to what it was during the disgusting Latin and Greek grammar? If the youngsters had become enraptured, if they sat quietly, mesmerized by the teacher's exciting presentation, what might Sir Alex say about the children's flawed nerves? We'd remind him that children's neurology does not change by modifying the curriculum presented, though their behavior might change appreciably.

[Behaviors associated with ADHD] may be minimal or absent when the [child] is under strict control, is in a novel setting, is engaged in especially interesting activities, is in a one-to-one situation (e.g., the clinician's office), or while the child experiences frequent rewards for appropriate behavior.[96]

That seems interesting, don't you think? The question asks, maybe what happens in the classroom might *override* a child's genetic predisposition, like by presenting unique, interesting, rewarding activities a teacher might bring about a change in a child's ADHD-like behavior? It's just a question seeking a response.

"That could be true," an ADHD advocate might be quick to concede, but add the coin has a second side. When, for example, kids are

> engaged in self-directed, highly rewarding activities ... it is often hard to see any attention deficit at all. ... [However], in situations where someone else is in charge of the task, when the activities are rote and the work is challenging and requires restraint and self-control, things get really bad in a hurry.[97]

Let's make lemonade out of that caution. "Things get bad in a hurry" suggests that things can get good in a hurry as well, if, again, we make some adjustments. Always beneficial to stay on the positive side.

We know that children behave differently in the presence of different teachers, that many children eagerly attend and participate when taught by teachers who regularly present rewarding, exciting, challenging, and doable assignments. That possibility suggests that the presumed state of the children's nerves, what physician Crichton pointed to as causing the offending children twiddles, may be less important than the setting and the curriculum assigned to the children. Then this, too. Suppose the material presented to the offending youngsters didn't match their skill sets, resulting in a situation where the children had no chance to be successful with their studies, not unlike an adult who's forced by a spouse to listen to a 60-minute lecture on the historical peculiarities of the soy bean. Tough for kids (or their Moms or Dads) to get excited (and stay focused) when faced with that possibility, the problem hardly the children's corrupted biology.

Perhaps Sir Alex's wiggly children weren't neurologically impaired, perhaps what he observed during that brief session was not an example of children genetically or neurologically compelled to fidget, perhaps other factors were involved. That's not something physician Crichton would have ever considered, his perspective, not unlike many of today's medical people, narrowly centered on biology and neurological pathology.

But *we* can consider alternatives, and we can try out ideas to probe if there's an exception to a rule. In place of medication as the first intervention, we could retrain the teacher and modify the curriculum. We could even show the children the benefits earned from their own initiated self-control and attention to task. (We're talking about a "self-management" program.) We could use a little behavioral strategy and announce to the kids: "Hey, once we spend 10 minutes on our dry, disgusting Latin and Greek grammar, we can play some word games that will help you with writing and spelling. You can pass fun notes back and forth or play 'Hangman' for a few minutes, quietly please. Then we'll do ten more minutes of this laborious grammar, after which we'll get out the building blocks and work on our geometry for a short while before we hit the grammar button again."

(FYI: That's called "When…Then contingencies.")

> "Wait…wait buddy, hold on a minute. You lost your marbles? You're talking lala land. Some teachers will never change, and some curriculum, it'll always be ugly. "

> "Are either reason enough to declare a child disordered when what's disordered has nothing to do with the child? Wouldn't it be wise to try a few things before we turn to medication?"

> "Yeah, right, smart guy. I've been there-Ritalin when I was six. So what are you gonna do, build a new school system?"

Please see: <https://www.nytimes.com/2017/08/11/nyregion/mastery-based-learning-no-grades.html?smid=nytcore-ipad-share&smprod=nytcore-ipad>

THE MEDICAL MODEL'S ADHD

The medical model assumes that a child's underachieving, inattentive, impulsive behavior is caused by some neuro-biogenetic irregularity, though "No one knows exactly what causes ADHD."[98]

Advocates view ADHD as a *disorder* a child *has*, similar in kind to other childhood ailments such as measles or mumps. Rather than being caused by a virus, however, ADHD is thought to be caused by neurobiological and/or genetic defects, not by anything that happens within a child's environment, a point made by the following claims:

> [ADHD] … has many causes, but all of the known causes fall within the realm of neurology and genetics. We can rule out the social environment, such as bad parenting, intolerant teachers, the breakdown of the American

family, a decline in family values, excess amount of TV viewing or video games. ... There's no evidence ... that will substantiate them.[99]

Again,

ADHD ... is not the result [of] laziness or lack of motivation and discipline. It is not caused by poor parenting, poor teaching, too much television, or too much time spent on fast paced video or computer games. ... Environmental contributors to ADHD are not credible.[100]

And again,

According to the National Resource Center on ADHD, "there's no strong evidence that parenting style contributes to [a child's] attention-deficit *disorder.*"[101]

Not unexpectedly, somebody's gonna raise a hand and say, "Uhm, I'd like to disagree."

[P]arental responses [to a child's] difficult behavior patterns may well promote a continuation of such patterns. In other words, genes and biology play a ... role in indicators of ADHD, but parental reactions to such behavior patterns are pivotal in forging their continuation and escalation.[102]

The disparity is striking, the positions nearly polar opposites. How are we to account for such inconsistency? Three authorities say parents and the environment have nothing to do with ADHD, that its base is exclusively biogenetic. Yet Drs. Stephen Hinshaw and Richard Scheffler offer a contrary view. If you'll look closely, you'll see what's happening. Reading the first three authoritative statements, it's clear the authors consider ADHD unrelated to, and unaffected by, anything within a child's current environment. For them, ADHD is a condition like measles or other childhood physical illnesses, caused by something biologic. A child who doesn't mind, a child who acts impulsively, a child who doesn't attend to his teacher or his studies is *driven* to act that way by his genes and/or his neurology. He can't help himself, like when he sneezes and rubs his eyes when tree pollen runs high. That's precisely what Dr. Crichton believed when observing the fidgety children. In his judgment, the school children's (supposed) frazzled nerves did to them what heat does to Zea mays everta, popping corn. But our dissenters thought otherwise. Their words, minimally edited, offer their diverse point of view. "...[P]arental responses [to a child's] difficult behavior patterns may well promote a continuation of such patterns. In other words, genes and biology play a...role in *indicators* of ADHD, but parental reactions to such behavior patterns are *pivotal* in forging their continuation and escalation." (Emphases are mine.)

Drs. Hinshaw and Scheffler have suggested that ADHD, whatever anyone thinks it is, is not independent of a child's environment. That means Moms and Dads and teachers (and many others) affect what a child does, what Drs. Hinshaw and Scheffler correctly refer to as "indicators," what you and I call "behaviors," though "indicators" is a more impactful term.

Let's suggest that Moms and Dads and teachers are able to modify a child's behavior, perhaps supersede a child's presumed (but not confirmed) biological predisposition toward impulsivity and inattention by changing the child's environment. That's what Drs. Hinshaw and Scheffler are intimating, in my view. If parents/teachers can *inadvertently* foster ADHD-like behavior, then they can also *intentionally*, by design (and professional assistance), foster desired alternative behavior. Just think, parents and educators might even teach a child to monitor himself, and, further, help him learn to successfully modify his own actions. That places a more optimistic slant on this ADHD business, that unlike uncontrolled pollen-induced sneezing, perhaps a child can make some decisions about his own behavior.

"Q": If a child no longer exhibits what Drs. Hinshaw and Scheffler suggest are "indicators of ADHD," does the child still have ADHD? If your previously mentioned cousin no longer exhibits any indicators of pneumonia, does she still have pneumonia? With ADHD, much depends on how we choose to define it. Let's see what CHADD (Children and Adults with Attention-Deficit/Hyperactivity Disorder) has to say.

DEFINITION

Despite many medical doctors arguing that ADHD fails to meet the minimum standards required of an officially recognized medical disorder, CHADD, a "nationally recognized authority on ADD/ADHD" has adopted the following ADHD definition:

> Attention-deficit/hyperactivity disorder is a neurobiological disorder characterized by developmentally inappropriate impulsivity, inattention, and in some cases, hyperactivity.[103] An estimated 75 to 80 percent of variation in the severity of ADD/ADHD-traits is the result of genetic factors. Some studies place this figure at over 90 percent.[104]

CHADD's definition fits squarely within the medical model. It represents the paradigm used by most medical, psychological, and educational practitioners to discuss, designate, and/or diagnosis ADHD. It clearly views ADHD as a *disorder* that results from an irregularity that exists *within* the youngster, specifically within a child's neurobiology. The definition provides a list of symptoms, a proposed cause, and what CHADD considers the name of the disorder, ADHD. Adding the hypothesized genetic component, the ADHD chart appears thusly (Box 4.2).

Box 4.2   ADHD

Cause	Disorder	Symptoms
Neurobiological, genetic factors	ADHD	Inappropriate impulsivity, inattention, and hyperactivity

(FYI A: Definitions are only as good as their ability to clarify the terms or concepts in question. Definitions provide "an *exact* statement or description of the nature, scope, or meaning of something." If components of a definition are ambiguous, the definition is insufficient: if two people reading the same definition leave with different interpretations, the definition remains for them inadequate. CHADD's definition is burdened by many constructs, terms that individuals define differentially. "Impulsivity," for example, represents many different possible actions. Because of impulsivity's inherent ambiguity, conflicting evaluations are inevitable, an outcome particularly troublesome when a teacher or parent is asked to rate whether a child behaves "impulsively." (That's referencing the highly elastic standard barometer we spoke of earlier.) Since the diagnosis of ADHD is either totally dependent on people's ratings, and/or a diagnostician's subjective judgment, which nearly always includes those ratings, "false positives" are unavoidable.

(FYI: Claiming that an individual is disordered when s/he's not is a "false positive.")

Before we evaluate the veracity of CHADD's proposed genetic and/ or neurological foundations for ADHD, I need you to consider the decisive feature of ADHD's proposed definition, namely that a child's behavior must be "developmentally inappropriate" to be considered disordered.

That inclusion is an indispensable condition of a traditional ADHD diagnostic decision. To clarify, if a child's behavior is perceived to be "developmentally *appropriate*," then what the child is doing is seen as fine, and ADHD is not an issue. If the converse exists where the child's behavior is judged "developmentally *inappropriate*," then ADHD is, according to CHADD's definition, a possibility. Let's look at those issues a little closer. They're not as straightforward as they may first appear.

The term "developmental" refers to the child's "age," and the term "inappropriate" refers to someone's personal judgment about a child's exhibited behavior. "Inappropriate" carries a definite negative connotation. The behavior is considered "not suitable and/or improper." Whether or not the behavior is also perceived to be psychologically or physically "pathological" depends on one's training and background. Though the judgment would be entirely subjective, medical model people lean in that direction. Here's an example.

A 3-year-old's thumb sucking would rarely be seen as developmentally inappropriate, though the child's parent might think otherwise. (Most kids give up the habit around 3–4 years of age.) However, a 10-year-old child who sucks his thumb would, according to some, be exhibiting a "developmentally inappropriate" behavior. As obvious as that might appear, please know that some professionals would not use the term "developmentally inappropriate" to describe even the 10 year old's unexpected behavior. They'd see the behavior as something that for unknown reasons serves some purpose for the child. If requested, they might help the child acquire another "more acceptable" way to satisfy his need, the concept of disorder, however, unnecessary. Again, regarding ADHD *indicators*, developmentally *inappropriate* is a judgment call.

If a child is thought to have ADHD, similarly in kind to suggesting that a child has mumps, several factors require consideration. The behaviors, what medical model people call "symptoms," actions such as "impulsivity," must be spoken of or written about in precise language. Impulsivity is not data-level language. An observer does not see "impulsivity." S/he sees a child's actions, behaviors that may warrant a number of different analyses. (Observed behaviors, what can be counted, are at the "data level.") Suggesting a behavior is inappropriate requires that we have some standard against which to compare it. Without an acceptable standard, a dozen people seeing the same behavior might, because of their own experiences, judge it differently, some voting "inappropriate," others disagreeing. That's a serious problem.

(FYI B: We have no established developmental norms for "impulsivity," no standard from which to draw an empirical comparison, no guide that says how many times a child needs to leave his seat or blurt out an answer within a ten-minute period to be judged impulsive or hyper or whatever descriptive term one wishes to use. As such, the declaration that a child is behaving impulsively is based on an observer's interpretation.)

Summarizing, according to CHADD's definition, whether a child meets ADHD's definitional criteria depends on the child's behavior, the child's developmental age, and someone's personal judgment regarding the behaviors. Putting all three factors together, consider the following situation that involves age, behavior, and judgment.

(We're going to fictitiously reduce a 5-year-old child's age by six months. Watch what happens.) If we told an unwitting diagnostician who had recently judged a kindergarten child's behavior "developmentally *inappropriate*" that the child in question was only four and a half years of age rather than five, the diagnostician might recant, "Oh, then he's not ADHD. At four and a half, his behaviors are not developmentally inappropriate." S/he'd have come to that conclusion even though the behaviors and the context within which they occurred had remained unchanged. All we did was change the child's age. If we unkindly suggested the child was really 4 years and 9 months old, the diagnostician might catch our motive and shrug his/her shoulders, agreeing, "it's a subjective judgment." You won't find that outcome or dilemma with mumps, where age and an observer's interpretive slant are irrelevant to any diagnosis. A microscope verifies mumps' virus; not so ADHD. It's camera-shy. There's the subjectivity of ADHD.

We've learned from the previous chapter that age is a poor variable to use to declare how a child should behave. Unlike mumps, a child's environment significantly affects a child's behavior at all ages. If a child is said to be inappropriately impulsive or inattentive, based entirely on the child's behavior, that evaluative conclusion reflects both the bias of the evaluator, and equally important the possible influence of the child's environment. To the degree that interpretation is correct, suggesting that a child has any disorder based on what s/he does would be arguable, at the very least.)

DISORDER

Since nothing about ADHD is neutral, it's not surprising when an authority questions the very basic assumption that ADHD is an organic disorder. Understand, please, that the term "disorder" is a necessary component of the medical model, as much as a spine is to a skeleton. CHADD intentionally used the term in its definition, referring to ADHD as a "neurobiological disorder." I have no doubts the organization was instructed by one of its paid physicians to adopt the above definition that specified the term "disorder."

I suggest that the term "disorder," with respect to ADHD, is an unnecessary distraction. It sets the tone of a discussion, a discussion better served if the term "disorder" were absent from the conversation. Better we speak of a child's behavior in its context, thinking in terms of what purpose the child's behavior might serve, thinking also whether or not the child needed to learn an alternative behavior, the concept of disorder unnecessary throughout. Since we've yet to reach broad consensus regarding "attention-deficit's" foundational structure, the term "disorder" is decidedly premature. David Mechanic has spoken to this issue.

Dr. David Mechanic, Rutgers University professor, writing in Stephen Hinshaw and Richard Scheffler's "ADHD Explosion," likewise questioned the use of the term "disorder" when discussing ADHD. He explains:

> There is some truth to the [assertion that] ADHD is commonly viewed as a contested behavior, not a true disorder, serving the interests of schools in their need to maintain order, the pharmaceutical industry that seeks to sell as many drugs as possible, or the varying professions and clinicians who build their practices around treatment of these children. ...
>
> [Though] ADHD is one of the most common diagnosis of children and adolescents as they proceed through their school experiences, ... considerable debate continues about whether ADHD is a real disorder, a convenient way of describing some troubling behaviors, or a reflection of our society and culture and the way we organize schools and learning. ... How much of the expansion [of ADHD] is a real increase in disorder, a reflection of growing definitional boundaries, a consequence of the changing nature of schooling and the focus on testing, stresses on teachers, or a response to advocacy and marketing of treatments remains a major puzzle. ...
>
> There is, of course, enormous biological variability; what we choose to view as disorder is in many ways a social construction. ... One criterion for such a definition is harm: the behaviors ... in question are in some significant way impairing, leading to ... disruptions in function. ... But this is insufficient for calling a troubling behavioral pattern a disorder.[105]

CAUSE

(FYI: In prelude to examining what CHADD sees as *causing* the proposed ADHD disorder, it's necessary to consider briefly the semantics of the term "cause." It comes with definitive elements.)

The word "cause" is used sparingly in the hard sciences. The term invariably communicates more than is intended. *Verifying* cause requires tight research controls and multiple replications where end results do not vary. Claiming "cause" suggests an unequivocal answer's been found and one need not look any further when considering an important puzzle or question. That's a dangerous attitude given the ever-changing *ecological* world that's constantly throwing surprises our way. Consider today's running, petulant debate on climate change. Best we leave the term "cause" in the attic. ADHD advocates seem unfazed by the term's rigorous demands. They use it liberally with impunity as if the scientific community has provided them a free pass. They haven't.

We can easily avoid the deep potholes "cause" sets in our path (Box 4.3).

Box 4.3   ADHD

Cause
Neurobiological, genetic factors

Consider the following example. The statement "smoking *causes* lung cancer" is more media talk than that of good science. Some folks have a history of heavy cigarette smoking since their teens and do not suffer lung cancer as adults. The few exceptions to the assumed cause/effect algorithm mean that other variables besides inhaling nicotine are involved. "Cause," then, even under the stated conditions is best avoided in favor of a more accurate and useful phrase: **Contribute to...**

Asserting "cause" is particularly misplaced in the field of education. Self-regulating social scientists avoid the word "cause" and discuss instead relations among variables with phrases such as "associated with" and "contributes to." Returning quickly to our smoking example, conservative medical scientists are apt to say "smoke inhalation from cigarettes strongly *contributes* to lung cancer." They'd point out that there's an established link—or a strong correlation between cigarette smoking and lung cancer (and many other cancers). Links reported in the high 0.9s (where "1.0" is the maximum) is as close as anyone needs to know that smoking's not a good choice for anyone. Still, the term "cause" is ill-advised. It's easy for young people to deny as they watch their elders puff away. It's not by accident that Drs. Hinshaw and Scheffler avoided the term "cause" when they discussed the pivotal role parents play with respect to children's ADHD-like behaviors. Reread their brief statement and you'll see that "contribute to" is clearly present without it being spoken. Once more, consider what psychologist and ADHD advocate Russell Barkley suggested regarding ADHD and its *causes*:

> [ADHD] ... has many causes, but all of the known causes fall within the realm of neurology and genetics. We can rule out the social environment, such as bad parenting, intolerant teachers, the breakdown of the American family, a decline in family values, excess amount of TV viewing or video games. ... There's no evidence ... that will substantiate them.[106]

For multiple reasons, the term "cause" is misused. Foremost, ADHD is a shorthand, representative term; it represents what kids and adults do. That's its function. As you'll see, ADHD is not directly (or indirectly) measurable, no more so than impulsivity is directly measurable. Only something measurable can qualify as a possible "cause" or, for that matter, an "effect," what is also known as an "outcome" variable. In a practical setting, a child's observable, data-level behaviors, like the number of times a youngster gets out of his seat or blurts out an answer during a 10-minute class, would be acceptable outcome variables. The behaviors can be counted, and their occurrences can be increased or decreased and counted again. Leaving a seat or blurting an answer is *not* caused, however. The most that can be said is that teachers and parents (and the child's fellow prodding classmates) can influence their occurrence. As such, it's permitted to say that the behaviors are possible effects, possible outcomes, of that influence. ADHD, the acronym, can't be an acceptable outcome variable or a cause. It doesn't have the structure to serve as either.

Notice, however, the advantages for the term "contribute." Would you have a problem if I suggested that parents, teachers, family values, television, and video games (and countless other variables) *contribute* to a child's behavior, even ADHD-like behavior? Can't imagine you would. Can you even talk about ADHD without mentioning what a child does and what contributes to it? You can't; the behaviors are all any of us see, not genetics or neurology. In fact, before we finish this chapter, you'll read where some very prominent scientist/practitioners believe ADHD is *only* the child's behavior.

With that notion, consider the child's ADHD-like behavior in light of what Drs. Hinshaw and Scheffler suggested about the role of parents: "… Parental reactions to such behavior patterns are pivotal in forging [the] continuation and escalation [of ADHD indicators]." Give some thought to that view as we now look at ADHD's purported neurological and/or genetic roots. Having done so, perhaps you'll suggest that Box 4.4 needs another entry under what CHADD considers ADHD's "cause," where "contribute" would be more suitable.

Box 4.4   ADHD

Cause	*Disorder*
Neurobiological, genetic factors, (parental reactions)	ADHD

ADHD: Neurology

Presumption: ADHD is a neurobiological disorder.[107]

CHADD could hardly be faulted for selecting exclusively a medical explanation for a child's poor classroom behavior. As suggested, its paid medical consultants probably wrote the definition. Selectively interpreted history assured the medical perspective. Notice, please. Early historians drew from reports recounting behaviorally challenging school children who had been exposed to some degree to the encephalitis lethargica epidemic from 1917 to 1918 and the pandemic of influenza from 1919 to 1920. Physicians considered the correlation between the epidemics and the reported behavior problems as supportive evidence that connected the children's school problems with their presumed impaired biology. The logic is questionable, but it was their logic.

(FYI: While it's tempting to suggest that the pandemics affected or "caused" the children's school problems, such interpreted correlations, certain to be statistically weak, would allow room for alternative interpretations regarding the purported school problems' footing, including one that would suggest that the children's observed behavior problems would have occurred had there been no epidemics. I don't recall any relevant pandemics in my lifetime, though I've seen quite a few behavior-problem children. I can confirm that something besides the children's biology was operating.)

"Q": Is ADHD's foundation neurological, as has been claimed? As you'll see, the answer is emphatically "No" (one reason in particular will become evident when we look at the relationship between ADHD and genetics). Let's examine the neurology closer. With respect to the proposed neurological base, recall the following, please:

- Speculation gained support from the medical profession that whenever a disruptive classroom behavior pattern was observed, it likely reflected underlying damage to the child's brain.[108]
- A syndrome emerged, one that came to be known as the "brain-injured child syndrome," a term that would be amended to minimal brain damage (MBD).[109,110]
- In the 1960s, "minimal brain damage" would be further amended to "minimal brain dysfunction syndrome."[111]
- The term "damage" was removed because no recognized organic damage could be found.[112]

Thanks in part to the model set by Sir Alexander Crichton, medical doctors, when concerning themselves with ADHD, continue to presume the presence of underlying neurological conditions such as a child's "state of nerves," though today they refer to "faulty wiring," or "minimal brain damage/dysfunction (MBD). They've been given permission to do so. Recall that "whenever a disruptive classroom behavior pattern was observed, it was interpreted to reflect an underlying biological damage that had impaired a child's brain."[113] Even when brain damage could *not* be demonstrated, it, astonishingly, could be *presumed* to be present. Earlier research[114,115] approved the general practice to *infer* brain damage (and eventually ADHD) solely from *behavioral signs* without any neurological evidence of damage.[116] (Emphases are mine.)

(FYI: You may have noticed the tautological relationship. "The child's hyperactivity is caused by his improper brain-wiring." "How do you know his brain is wired improperly? I don't see any signs on the x-ray." "You don't have to see it on x-rays. Just look at his hyperactivity.")

MBD[117]

"Some professionals believe all children [who exhibit poor classroom achievement] suffer from a dysfunction of the central nervous system. ... In cases in which actual evidence of brain damage *cannot* be shown, ... the term 'minimal brain dysfunction' is sometimes used, especially by physicians who assume that the child's brain does not function properly.[118] Other physicians are quick to point out that "minimal brain damage is an invalid designation. It doesn't exist."[119] In particular, psychiatrist Roger D. Freeman expanded his rejection of MBD to include a most salient point, his view for us significant. He stated, "There is simply no such thing as minimal brain damage." He then expanded his position and suggested cogently, "Every time the designation is used there is a chance that it will simply mask another [variable],"[120] one that might be contributing to a problem that we've asserted is caused by a biological error. "Mask another variable" easily prompts us to recall a child without sufficient skills who was required to trudge through his teacher's dry and disgusting Latin and Greek grammar. Unfortunately, the concept of "mask another variable" didn't encourage Sir Alex to consider trading his diagnostic MBD, i.e., "state of nerves," for what he witnessed first hand: the problematic curriculum. Some of today's physicians asked to evaluate a struggling school child are likewise reluctant to reconsider their neurologically based explanations.[121] Like Crichton, they've been away from grade school for a long time.

There's no denying that the brain is a convenient source point for an unending number of explanations. It's full of astounding possibilities, it still hides most of its remarkable secrets, and where better to place responsibility for a child's underachievement and inattentiveness if we want to keep a scientific challenge at bay. Consider the proposed educational disorders that have no obvious organic structure or medical markers, such as dyslexia, dyscalculia, dysgraphia. Just summon the spirit of minimal brain damage as an explanation for a child's achievement struggles. We can deny MBD's existence but we cannot refute it. In many medical circles, it always wins the debate, not because it's correct, but because it requires little thought. We speak as if we know all the workings of this extraordinarily complex two-sided organ that is our executor. Quite naive of us.[122]

There are certainly some structural differences that brain imaging shows— this part of the brain is a little smaller than normal and that part is a bit bigger. However, brain imaging is a snapshot of the brain's structure that is taken in a fraction of a second and tells you nothing about whether a [child] has ADD/ADHD [or manifests ADHD-like behaviors]. Attention deficit hyperactivity disorder is not a structural [physical] problem in the brain.[123]

The medical journals are littered with the remains of discarded theories that purport to explain restlessness in children as a symptom of a disease. ... What is remarkable here is not the series of failures to find a biological cause but the tenacity with which this line of investigation continues to be pursued.[124]

There is some evidence of cortical thinning in brain structures related to attention which *may* result in less efficient cognitive processes.[125] (Researcher added emphasis to qualify the less efficient claim)

The 1998 Consensus Development Conference, held by the US National Institutes of Health, came to this conclusion: "[W]e do not have an independent, valid test for ADHD, and there are no data to indicate that ADHD is due to a brain malfunction."[126]

It seems we're plagued by the lure of simple answers. Notice the following.

Brain imaging studies have revealed that, in youth with ADHD, the brain matures in a normal pattern but is delayed, on average, by about 3 years.[127]

Though an easy statement to make, one that would be accepted in most circles without criticism, it suffers from two serious failings. The lesser of the two relates to "brain maturity," where a quick review of literature reveals the following:

- Speaking at least of the adolescent brain, "very little can be extrapolated from the science to illuminate individual behavior. The research simply does not allow one to measure the maturity of the individual brain."[128]
- The frontal lobes, home to key components of the neural circuitry underlying "executive functions" such as planning, working memory, and impulse control are among the last areas of the brain to mature; they may not be fully developed until halfway through the third *decade* of life.[129] (Emphasis mine.)
- Less clear is whether neuroimaging, at present, helps to inform age-based determinations of maturity.[130]

- The ability to designate an adolescent as "mature" or "immature" neurologically is complicated by the fact that neuroscientific data are continuous and highly variable from person to person; the bounds of "normal" development have not been well delineated.

To the more serious problem with the study, the authors suggested, "the brain matures in a normal pattern but is delayed in youth with ADHD." That declaration assumes ADHD is a diagnosable entity, one that makes it easy to distinguish between a group of children with ADHD and one without ADHD. That assumption is without merit, as you'll see when we look at how ADHD is identified. For now, it's sufficient to say that the construct "ADHD" does not lend itself to such exacting differentiation. The best the researchers could claim, and stay within the boundaries of scientific propriety, would limit the message to something like "human brains mature on different schedules," and "the behavioral timetables of children (and adolescents) vary considerably." Neither statement says much that's substantive, but both are honest.

Though the claim has been made that "ADHD-related problems are widespread throughout the brain,"[131] the assertion requires that we know specifically what problems the author referenced, what was not mentioned, and, more challenging, how those apparent school-related problems, underachievement, inattentiveness, show themselves within brain tissue, a significant feat that would require that both leave an organic footprint. We must reconcile the statement that ADHD problems are widespread throughout the brain against the disclosure that

> "...findings do not allow diagnosis of ADHD via brain scans. The variation across individuals is simply too great, the brain is unfathomably complex, and the field's knowledge of its workings is still rudimentary."

The same researchers who acknowledge those accurate limitations have expressed with hopeful anticipation, "Perhaps some forms of ADHD will one day be known to have a particular brain 'signature,' but for now diagnosis must be based on observations of behavior patterns and thorough clinical judgment."[132]

I'm afraid the researchers are headed toward inevitable disappointment. Catching a glimpse of ADHD's signature can never happen.

No one found it under a microscope. No one discovered it from a lab test. It doesn't show up in urine or blood. You can't find it anywhere in the body.[133] (Mary Ann Block, DO, Osteopathic Physician and Author)

ADHD was never discovered or validated by demonstration of a confirmatory physical (including chemical) abnormality. Rather, ADHD was invented in-committee at the American Psychiatric Association in 1980.[134]

No matter how we decode ADHD, the acronym possesses *no* neurobiological mark.

ADHD has no physiological markers. There are no physical findings, no laboratory tests, no x-rays or psychological tests that alone can be used to make the diagnosis of ADHD,[135] no neurological markers[136] available to physicians or psychologists for determining whether a child has ADHD.[137]

[C]riticisms that there's no biological marker for the disorder [are] lame. If you're saying that we don't understand ADHD down to the level of molecules and cells and proteins within the brain, well, that's true. But that's true of many disorders in medicine and in all of psychology.[138]

ADHD can't leave its signature, figurative or otherwise. The problem is, has been, and will always be ADHD's bony skeleton—it *doesn't* have one.

People speak of ADHD as if you could take it into a lab where in seconds you'd have on digital film its face and its form. How casual we are with such grand-sounding statements like "[T]he overall brain volume of individuals with ADHD is somewhat smaller than that of non-ADHD individuals."[139] A reader of such a claim can't help but believe we have at our disposal a definitive, reliable measure that differentiates one remarkably heterogeneous group (individuals *with* ADHD) from another remarkably heterogeneous group (individuals *without* ADHD) as if the two groups were as discrete as

- Group A ≥ 1828.9 millimeters tall
- Group B < 1828.8 millimeters tall

or as if ADHD's identification was as simple as psychiatrist Paul Wender's notion:

Fidgeting and foot movements ... are common signs of hyperactivity ... so much so that [people] can usually be diagnosed in the waiting room by a knowledgeable receptionist. ... I'm seriously entertaining the possibility that this foot movement may be a biological marker for ADHD.[140]

One ponders where within what group of cells we will find the imprint of psychiatrist Wender's fidgety foot movements or Johnny Jones' disruptive classroom antics? ADHD has no such reliable neurological marker and no neurological underpinning. ADHD is psychiatry's chosen name, its darling was how it was once described. It is psychiatry's convenient construct that makes conversation easier, hardly an attribute to celebrate.

> Psychiatry has never validated ADHD as a biologic entity, so their fraud and their misrepresentation is in saying to the parents of the patients in the office… that this…diagnosis is, in fact, a brain disease.[141]

It is curious that we've spent so much time over these past decades debating the alleged neurological basis of a child's obstructive behavior when, in fact, whether there is or isn't such a neurological base is irrelevant to any strategy we might choose on behalf of the child. The child's counter-behavior is sufficient evidence to set strategies in motion. It seems we're more concerned with keeping ADHD's flag waving than providing the child more functional behaviors. That's our attention deficit, not the child's.

ADHD: Genes

Presumption: "Heredity is the most common cause of ADHD."[142]

It is said that:

- ADHD tends to run in families. Studies have shown certain genetic characteristics that occur with high frequency in families where one or more family member has ADHD.[143]
- When ADHD-style behaviors persist beyond toddlerhood, at levels that are extreme given the person's age, they reflect genetically transmitted vulnerability.[144]
- Research suggests that ADHD is largely a genetic disorder.[145]
- The polygenetic nature of ADHD indicates that multiple genes jointly contribute to the development of ADHD with each having a modest effect on the overall risk.[146]
- Family and twin studies of ADHD demonstrate a high heritability, estimated to be around 70–80% from twin studies.[147]

Taken at face value, a solid link between ADHD and genetics appears to be established. Google "Genetics and ADHD" and you'll be hard-pressed to find any opposition to the purported relationship between ADHD and genetics, a relationship so assured that one of its confident proponents suggested that "Genes account for some 80% of ADHD."[148]

Skeptics do exist. Lydia Mary Furman, MD, pediatrician at Cleveland's Children's Hospital, argued concisely: "Evidence for a genetic or neuroanatomic cause of ADHD is insufficient. ADHD is unlikely to exist as an identifiable disease."[149] We're further instructed,

That personality in general, and ADD personality in particular, has a genetic component is highly likely. ... The error of biological psychiatry is in making too much of this connection. Most of the studies that show ... links [between the two] suffer from methodological flaws that make it difficult to entirely separate the effects of family heredity from those of family environment.[150]

It's been said that "most of the reason for high level focus and self-regulation of some people (and the lack of such abilities in others) is found in the genes rather than child-rearing practices or environments. The lesson here is that even if a trait or condition shows strong heritability, environments still matter."[151]

In the journal *Biological Psychiatry*, Harvard Medical School professor David Pauls wrote that a complex genetic disorder is one that does not follow strict patterns of inheritance. He suggested that complex disorders "are caused by a combination of a number of genetic, environmental and stochastic [randomly determined] factors [that] ... lead to similar if not identically looking outcomes."[152]

Despite a wealth of evidence supporting the involvement of genetics, very few studies have withstood replication. [G]enome-wide association studies found no significant associations, suggesting that any gene variant for ADHD must have a small effect.[153,154]

[Say] parents who were psychologically disturbed brought up psychological[ly] disturbed children. This would not be genetic. ... Not everything that runs in families is genetic. And how strongly something runs in a family doesn't tell us if it is transmitted genetically or through learning. All the offspring of Chinese-speaking parents speak Chinese—this is 100 percent learned. A fairly small fraction of the children of a red-headed parent have red hair—and having red hair is a trait that is hereditarily transmitted. The problem is [always] one of separating nature [genetics] from nurture [environmental learning].[155]

Published studies have tested for an association between ADHD and 27 different candidate genes. ... 14 of these candidate genes appear to account for a relatively small proportion of the variance in ADHD symptoms, suggesting that none are likely to be necessary or sufficient to cause ADHD.[156]

Extensive time and professional energy has focused on substantiating a neurobiological and/or genetic bond to ADHD. As many previous citations have testified, the results have been disappointing.[157]

In a moment of brash optimism, we learned,

In 2010, the British Broadcasting Company (BBC) announced boldly: "The first direct evidence of a genetic link to attention deficit hyperactivity disorder has been found." Anita Thapar, professor of child and adolescent psychiatry, Cardiff University, expressed her hope "that these findings will help overcome the stigma associated with ADHD. Too often, people dismiss ADHD as being down to bad parenting or poor diet. ... Now we can say with confidence that ADHD is a genetic disease and that the brains of children with this condition develop differently to those of other children."[158]

It's been suggested that primary prevention and early intervention techniques are impossible without the full understanding of ADHD's etiology. It's been further stated that if a genetic connection could be made, informed parents would be able to lessen or even reverse the effects established by the child's genetic makeup.

Psychologist Erik Willcut suggested that if a perinatal screening [around the time of childbirth] revealed significant genetic susceptibility to ADHD, parents could be provided with education and consultation regarding child behavior management techniques that may help to minimize or eliminate the impairment caused by symptoms of ADHD if their infant were to develop such symptoms.[159]

According to the psychologist, identification of specific genes responsible for ADHD would allow the formulation and distribution of new and better drugs for children.

Psychologist Willcut continued: "By providing a better understanding of underlying pathophysiology, molecular genetic techniques will inform the development of tertiary pharmacological or psychosocial treatments that directly target the specific neurophysiological mechanisms that are compromised in ADHD. (The assertions demand a counterview. Please see "critique.")[160]

In 1998, Russell Barkley echoed Willcut's viewpoint: "The day is not far off when genetic testing for ADHD may become available and more specialized medications may be designed to counter the specific genetic deficits of the children who suffer from it."[161]

Much is riding on the assumption that ADHD *and* genotypes are highly correlated. Researchers want to know if ADHD-like behaviors are exhibited given a child's unique genotype—the child's genetic constitution provided mostly by his or her parents. (*Mostly* because DNA mutations can occur randomly in egg or sperm cells, or after conception in an early embryo.)[162]

If a particular gene or constellation of genes shows up when a child consistently exhibits a counterproductive set of behaviors, if the gene or set of genes is absent when a child behaves opposite to the counterproductive behaviors, and if it can be established that *no* environment variables contributed to the child's behaviors, then evidence gathered might hint at a relationship between the child's genetic makeup and the child's *behavioral manifestations*. If the findings can be replicated multiple times, further evidence would be added to the hypothesis that there exists a relationship between the child's genes and the exhibited *behaviors*.

As solid as the above may sound, it's not that clean or simple. Suppose the same child exhibits both productive and nonproductive behaviors the same day, perhaps within the same hour? Suppose the child exhibits the nonproductive behavior while struggling with Latin and Greek grammar, with multiplication tables, with the genetics of the drosophila fruit fly, but not with Harry Potter? Not with Copernicus? Not with quantum mechanics, or the life cycle of killer whales? Are we talking about genes? With that amount of behavioral variability within minutes? Not likely. We already know what psychologist Barkley said about genes and ADHD: "Genes account for some 80% of ADHD." Before we look at what geneticists say, an essential point regarding genes needs to be clarified.

(FYI: Despite all the claims that genes are responsible for a child's ADHD, it's *not* ADHD that's correlated with a child's genes. That correlation is between a child's *phenotype* and his/her genes. (Actually, the potential relationship is even more diluted. Said correctly, the correlation is between an evaluator's *perception* of a child's phenotype and the child's genes.))

What is "phenotype?" In plain language, a child's behavior. More technically, "the set of observable characteristics [behaviors] resulting from the interaction of a child's genotype with the environment." Genotype? That's an individual's innate genetic identity.

Professor Barkley's remarkable statement that genes account for some 80% of ADHD is factually and semantically inaccurate. Once again, ADHD is the name psychiatry chose to use. It's a convenient construct that represents what a child does. That's its role, like "height" represents inches from a person's toes to her crown, and "weight" represents numbers that register on an applicable scale. Before one can even challenge Barkley's extraordinary declaration, the man's statement *must* read, "genes account for 80% of a child's *phenotype*." In other words, genes account for 80% of a child's selected, directly observable behavior, his/her actions: doesn't answer questions, talks too much, runs around too much, doesn't finish assignments, is inattentive and disruptive, cries when corrected.

Regardless of the chosen behavioral outcome measures, such a claim that genes account for 80% of a child's behavior would be impossible to verify, a child's contributing (and confounding) environment ever-present from birth." As pointed out moments ago, "The problem is [always] one of separating nature [genetics] from nurture [environmental learning]."

More to the point, no self-regulating researcher would ever suggest that eye-popping degree of relationship between genes and a child's school/home-related behavior, even if several of the behaviors were "ADHD-like." The figure 80%, representing how much variance (influence) genes have on a child's behavior, implies that Moms and Dads and the rest of a child's environment have had minimal effect on the youngster's everyday conduct. You think? Give your parents a buzz and get their take, whether they were just twiddling their toes and smelling the rubarb while you were being led around your world by your genes.

When you see how such genetic-ADHD attribution research is conducted, you'll understand why the claim is untenable. In the name of genetics, we're prone to taking lots of liberties.

Claims that genes account for 80% of ADHD are based mostly on reported findings from researchers who investigated the presence or absence of ADHD-like behaviors within the population of monozygotic twins (identical twins) and dizygotic twins (fraternal twins), some of the children raised by natural parents, some by adoptive parents.[163] On the surface, the research is straightforward. Offering you the short version, the gene-attribution researchers do something like the following.

- They identify two kids, one purportedly exhibiting ADHD-like behaviors, one who does not, the differentiation according to teachers or parents who judged the children's behaviors. Blood is drawn from the children and genes are checked.

- Researchers identify identical twins and fraternal twins, some purportedly exhibiting ADHD-like behaviors, some without, again according to teachers or parents who judged the two children. Blood is drawn and genes are checked.
- Researchers identify twins separated and raised by different families, some exhibiting ADHD-like behaviors, some who do not, according to the individual evaluators who judged the two children. Blood is taken and genes are checked.

The researchers spend roughly an hour on the phone with one of the parents of an evaluated child to gain family medical and mental health history. Once researchers have the family history, they examine blood samples and look for a DNA pattern that's unique for children thought to have ADHD, and children thought not to have ADHD, yet again, the ADHD component as judged by the parent or teacher evaluator.

The manner in which the children were judged does raise some questions. Since researchers rarely, if ever, see the kids, they're totally reliant on the evaluators who report the children's behaviors. Each solicited evaluator is expected to describe the child's behavior and its history, precisely, objectively, honestly. The researcher assumes the evaluators do so. In actual practice, the information provided by the evaluators may be valid and reliable, or it may not be. The researcher seldom, if ever, knows.)

Summarizing, for genetic/ADHD-attribution research to yield meaningful findings, researchers must have control over all critical variables, an accurate measurement of genes, and a measure of ADHD-like behaviors. Stating the obvious,

- We can't legitimately claim an association between genes and ADHD if one or both components are not directly observable and measurable.
- We can't legitimately claim an association between genes and ADHD if the effects of the child's influential environment on the child's behavior are unknown.
- Likewise, we can't claim an association between genes and a child's *phenotype* if the effects of the child's influential environment are unknown.

The studied subjects aren't little white mice, where their environments are small cages over which the researchers have total control. With genetic/ADHD-attribution research, the interactions between parents and kids at home are significant factors, their extent, much less their specifics, mostly unknown to the researchers. May I remind you once again of Drs. Hinshaw's and Scheffler's admonition: "Parental responses to a child's difficult behavior patterns may well promote a continuation of such patterns. ...Parental reactions to such behavior patterns are pivotal in forging their continuation and escalation."

A child's ADHD-like behavior, what we see a child do, has multiple contributors. Many genetic/ADHD-attribution researchers are aware of environmental contributors, and are quick to acknowledge that such contributors affect a child's behavior, what represents one of their critical research variables. By that awareness, they know that their research findings will be affected by variables over which they have no control: what happens in the classroom between teachers and students, and what happens at home between parents and their child. That's an open invitation to chance, what will impact their results, and challenge their conclusions. When you see the results of their genetic/ADHD attribution research, you might have a clearer understanding of how those results came about.

Research Issues Geneticists know what they're doing. Their subject matter, genes, lends itself to direct observation and verification. Consensus with respect to which gene is being studied rarely presents a problem.

Such is not the case with ADHD. "Studies differed considerably with regard to [the] diagnostic criteria, rating scales [and] interview methods" used to assess what the researchers considered to be ADHD.[164]

- If the child judged himself or herself, that could present a serious problem.
- If the only judge was the parent, that could present a serious problem.
- If the only judge was the child's teacher, that could be a serious problem.

Cautionary notes from genetic researchers[165]:

- The use of single-rater assessment (and single measures) can result in unacceptable measurement error variance, which in turn can adversely influence power to detect susceptibility genes.

- Uncertainty about validity and measurement suggests that molecular genetic studies of ADHD should not rely on maternal reports alone.
- Heritability estimates are highly variable. Given these variable findings, together with the problems of using a single rater, using teacher reports alone for molecular genetic studies of ADHD is not recommended.
- It needs to be borne in mind that if single raters are used, studies based on maternal reports and studies based on teacher ratings may yield different findings.
- Data cast doubts about the utility of self-reports of ADHD in molecular genetic studies.
- It is less straightforward deciding how exactly to combine data from parents and teachers, and different research groups may integrate data from different informants differently to yield categorical clinical diagnoses. There is even greater uncertainty as to how best to integrate scores from different reporters.

Because of these differences, particularly the erratic ADHD diagnostic criteria, and how the data were collected, the following essential question must be asked: "What were the genetic/ADHD-attribution studies measuring when researchers had parents, guardians, and teachers describe a child, or more often fill out forms used to assess a child's ADHD-like behaviors?" Two critical variables are always involved in genetic/ADHD research. If we can't accurately measure a child's genes, we have no study. If we can't accurately measure ADHD, we have no study. If we can't accurately measure and account for the interactional effects of the child and his/her environment, we have no study. If the data are sketchy with no external experimental controls, we may have a study, though a poor one.

Fact: *None* of the published genetic/ADHD-attribution studies measured ADHD. All, using varying methods, collected and evaluated tabulated scores reflecting a child's *behavior*, the information obtained from unsupervised observations, and/or answers on paper/pencil questionnaires, checklists or rating scales filled out by parents, teachers, relatives, and/or guardians.

Fact: *None* of the questionnaires, checklists, or rating scales measured ADHD. All questionnaires, checklists, and rating scales provided researchers minimal samples of a child's behavior as seen and interpreted through the *eyes* of evaluators: parent, teacher, relatives, and/or guardians.

The data were collected with few, if any, experimental controls, the results with an unknown degree of random error.

"[P]arents themselves may vary in their perceptions of the child's behavior depending on their levels of stress, exhaustion, or skill in behavior management."[166] "Mothers tend to over report, compared with teachers,"[167] and "mothers with problems [e.g., depression] tend to report more behavior problems in their children, problems not independently confirmed."[168]

Special educators, for example, "are more tolerant of ADD-type behavior compared to regular classroom teachers."[169] Even co-teachers who experience the same hour and full day in front of the same children differ markedly in their views. Drs. Hinshaw and Scheffler pointed out that "[c]ompared to a teacher untrained in dealing with problem behavior, a particularly warm and responsive teacher may rate the child less problematic."[170] Contrasting judgments among teachers produce different checklist tallies,[171] resulting in divergent, inconsistent numbers presented to the physician or psychologist— one teacher claiming a child's high behavior frequencies, only to be contradicted by a second or third teacher.

With genetic studies, selecting, defining, and identifying the children's behaviors (their phenotype) that fit under the umbrella of ADHD remains a controversial issue. Counting and rating those behaviors has proven difficult. Agreements between parents and teachers (the evaluators) correlate around 0.3,[172] a very *low* rating. (A reading of 0.3 means that teachers and parents who observe the same scene either don't agree on what they're seeing or don't use the same tallying system when filling out questionnaires, checklists, and rating scales. That's called experimental error.) Problems arise with genetic studies when differences in rater assessments reflect sources other than the ADHD trait of interest.[173] That's also called experimental error. Experimental error raises serious doubts about any drawn conclusions.

Who are these essential individuals required to collect, recall, and report vital data to the genetic researchers? They're ordinary folks, moms, dads, grandmas, aunts, teachers with difficult children/pupils of their own, all who, during data collection, must remain neutral and objective, who must report only what's true, accurate, and meaningful, who must avoid reporting either what they think a researcher might want them to report, or what they think will get them what *they* want.

Most often, these evaluators receive no formal training that might increase their accurate observing and recording, and often not as much as a brief pre-evaluation personal interview. They know they're to describe *their* child's behavior. They know that ADHD is the topic in question. They know what may result from their answers, that their child may be diagnosed ADHD and thereby become a candidate for medication and/or school accommodations. That awareness may contaminate the procedures, affecting a researcher's results and his or her conclusions. Many experienced physicians expect such biased reports.

"Teacher reports almost invariably come back as citing the behaviors that would warrant a diagnosis, a decision [physician Anderson] called more economic than medical."[174] —Michael Anderson, MD Pediatrician.

ENLISTING EVALUATORS

Diagnosing ADD over the telephone is a growing trend in child psychiatry research. In ... published studies, children were diagnosed with ADD after evaluators spoke only to their mothers on the telephone,[175] and recent researchers relied on postal questionnaires where parents [under unknown conditions] filled out forms that judged their children ADHD.[176]

Without having met the evaluators, researchers ask stressed parents, (and exhausted teachers) to fill out questionnaires, checklists, and rating scales that can challenge the most highly qualified, objective professionals. Most often,

- The evaluators' reliability is unknown.
- Their ability to judge behaviors and score them accurately is unknown.
- Their emotional state is unknown.
- Their intentions, agendas, aspirations are unknown.

First-year psych graduate students understand what's termed "Respondent Bias," where reported results are influenced less by the variables being observed and more by variables that affect those who perform the observations.

Genetic/ADHD-attribution researchers believe these folks will do a fine job. Researchers never know if they do a fine job—or if they skewed their data. Researchers might conclude that errors, if any, will wash out, meaning they balance themselves, some good, some not so good, added together equals neutral. They might use a statistical manipulation where they include within their analysis room for error without ever knowing the degree of error. The researchers might accept the numbers produced by the evaluators and assume *in numeris veritas*, i.e., truth in numbers.

When genetic/ADHD-attribution researchers make cold telephone calls with little to no knowledge of the family's dynamics, the acquired data are left more to chance than to planned controls. Without vetting the evaluator, the researcher has no prior knowledge of the teacher's (or parent's) ability to score accurately the child's behavior. Are the people interviewed *wanting* an ADHD diagnosis? Are they *ready* to exaggerate a child's problems to gain that diagnosis? There are benefits involved. Without a pre-interview (and often even with a pre-interview), a teacher's or parent's agenda, if one exists, remains a mystery, rendering its effects on the data a wild card.

Numbers derived from the instruments are assumed accurate even though no safeguards are put in place to warrant the assumption. Researchers seize the numerical scores. Once the numbers find their place on paper, and the paper finds itself in marked folders, the data not only acquire life, they acquire authenticity. The parents and teachers, whoever they were, however they scored a child, no longer elicit concern. The data are in hand. They are assumed accurate representations.

In one study, parents who were asked to decide whether their child was ADHD were recruited by college students (who earned extra credit) enrolled in an intro to psych class. The students were directed to "find parents of 'normal' children ages 5-17 years old.")[177] The study's authors reported that the subjects were obtained "primarily through convenience," an honest admission. The authors, however, made no mention of assessing the parent's qualifications to evaluate (diagnose) their children. The authors did share the following disclaimer: "[A] potential limitation [of the study was] using parent reports in the evaluation of childhood disorders."[178] That's a significant statement. The study's most important data come from the parents. The researchers reported their results, and the results were believed.

In studies like the one mentioned, researchers reveal such limitations with the readers of the research papers. Not all researchers do. If a researcher chooses to say nothing in the face of serious shortcomings, instead choosing to make claims without qualification, the study borders on unethical. Disclaimers are part of sound research. Reviews like the following make it easy to judge the value of published results.

- The earliest twin study on the heritability of hyperactivity was performed by Willerman in 1973.[179] This study used a volunteer sample and questionnaires of uncertain validity. The fear was expressed that volunteers might falsify results.
- Different measurement instruments assessed the same underlying behavioral construct. ... Rater-specific variance [discrepancy] was found for both parent and teacher data.
- Studies (reviewed) differed considerably with regard to the diagnostic criteria, rating scales or interview methods; their addressing environmental risk factors also differed.[180]

I located an extensive review of multiple studies (called a "meta-analysis") involving genetic/ADHD-attribution research. The review listed the various studies' findings along with their shortfalls to counterbalance, when necessary, what researchers may have stated or implied about their questionable, positive findings. The following are some abridged examples of noted weaknesses:

- The studies need to be improved and replicated.
- Failed to replicate the results.
- Unable to replicate the results.
- Found no evidence of a relationship between ADHD and ... [genetic component].
- Conflicting results reported.
- Results are inconsistent.
- Although there have been many reports supporting a positive association, there are also negative findings.
- Contradictory findings noted.
- No relationship found between ADHD and ... .
- No clear evidence has been reported to support an association between ADHD and ... .
- There is more than one report with contradictory findings.

The most frequent finding throughout the 13 pages of reviews was the absence of consistent results when evaluating the association (correlation) between ADHD and its presumed genetic foundation. The review's authors had little option but to state: "To date, the findings from genetic studies in ADHD have been somewhat inconsistent and disappointing."[181] Part of the problem? The studies *weren't* measuring anything but evaluators' *perceptions* of behaviors exhibited by their child, or some-one else's child.

> Although twin studies [claim] that ADHD is a highly heritable condition, molecular genetic studies suggest that the genetic architecture of ADHD is complex. The handful of genome-wide linkage and association scans that have been conducted thus far show divergent findings and are, therefore, *not conclusive*. Many of the candidate genes reviewed are compelling but available data are sparse and inconsistent.[182] (Emphases are mine)

The propensity to make positive claims only to temper those very claims was a common occurrence among researchers who investigated the genetic/ADHD relationship. One can't help but believe the researchers were determined to find a relationship because they wanted one to exist. The following is a classic example of the two steps forward and the three steps back.

> "A more direct method of examining the heritability of ADHD is to study twins: the extent to which monozygotic twins are more concor-dant for ADHD than dizygotic twins can be used to compute the degree to which variability in ADHD in the population can be accounted for by genes (i.e., heritability)."[183]

But the same author pointed out:

> "That environmental factors do play a significant role in the etiology of ADHD is unquestionable."

The author, after claiming that "Attention-deficit hyperactivity disorder (ADHD) is one of the most highly heritable childhood psychiatric disor-ders," was quick to temper his enthusiasm when pointing out that,

> "although [twin] studies are theoretically compelling, replication of these results has been inconsistent."[184]

After reading the positives and their turn-about qualifiers, you can't help feeling like you're caught in a hotel's revolving door, inside one moment, outside in the cold the next. This begs the question, "What did the researchers really find?"

> "Meta-analyses have produced more reliable results, but the associations identified to date account for only a *small percentage* of the genetic compo-nent of ADHD."[185] (Emphases mine.)

There's one certainty in all the ADHD-genetic attribution studies: ADHD was *not* studied. Questionnaires, checklist scores, and subjective ratings provided by evaluators were studied, though with extraordinarily loose controls. Research claims were based on statistical analyses, not direct observation of any child. If you're not aware of this, a good statistician can prove the earth is flat.

What did those scores obtained from evaluators and used by the researchers really reflect? No one knows, not the researchers, not the evaluators. Anyone can make all manner of claims, but when you run a mix of variables (uncontrolled observations) through a statistical blender, you may lose the central feature you were studying. Look at the ingredients: stressed adults and difficult children and researchers watching indirectly from afar.

Conclusion A: We have *no* studies that compare genes and ADHD. We're still arguing over what ADHD is, much less how to measure it. Rather, we have great numbers of studies that compare children's genes with how evaluators fill out forms, forms that report what kids *do*, or more often what the kids once *did*—last week, last month, or last year. When an evaluator fills out a form, s/he is asked to consider the child over extensive time, not just yesterday or last night when the child was difficult. (How well an exasperated parent or teacher can disassociate herself from recent emotional strain brought on by the child she's now judging is not known.) This need for recollections calls into question an evaluator's perceptions, emotions, attention, and memory skills, important variables if those same people are the conveyers of the data that will affect the research studies' findings.

Conclusion B: The *most important subjects* in studies that attempt to correlate genes and what we think of as ADHD aren't the children being observed, but the evaluators who are doing the observing. If the evaluators aren't accurate and precise in their counting and reporting, if they're not objective but instead are pressured by their own needs, researchers are provided questionable or faulty data. If researchers choose to ignore the strong possibility of faulty data, they'll likely draw faulty conclusions.

Conclusion C: What's lacking in genetic/ADHD attribution research are phenotypes inalterably driven by a child's genes, in the same way a child's illness is produced inalterably by an identified biological variant, a bacterium, for example. If you have the biological variant, you have the illness. No equivocation. If you have the ADHD anomalous gene, you have the ADHD-phenotype. That's what we want. In gene research, as it relates to the medical model's ADHD, we're talking about "endophenotypes."

> The search for an appropriate way to define psychiatric phenotypes ... [a child's observable behaviors] is increasingly recognized to be of crucial importance for understanding the genetic basis of both child and adult psychiatry.[186] The characteristics of potentially valuable endophenotypes ... are clear—they should be measurable reliably, both over time and by different observers.[187]

"Endophenotypes"[188] are observable, measurable characteristics (behaviors) thought to be *genetic* in origin. "Genetic in origin" is the *key* attribute. Endophenotypes represent a child's inherent temperament.

- They're the way children are *predisposed* to behave.
- They're what are genetically driven, innate, that which lend children their very special character and uniqueness.

Endophenotypes are *not* learned. That's a second key attribute. Endophenotypes are members of their own elite, private club. Without ADHD endophenotypes, there's *no* authentic, reliable ADHD/genetic connection.

> Drs. Alexis Wood and Michael Neale have noted that "there is a lack of consensus regarding the necessary and sufficient steps for empirically validating a [behavior] as a suitable candidate for an ADHD endophenotype."[189]

Since we have no empirically verified behavioral candidates that qualify as endophenotypes, the acronym ADHD fails to represent any universally acceptable behavior that can be said to confirm ADHD and its genetic foundation. All studies seeking to confirm that ADHD is a genetic disorder are compromised from the start by their need to possess a *valid* measure of ADHD. Without that measure, we have what we should expect: inconclusive and often conflicting research results. Though Dr. Barkley claimed genes constitute 80% of ADHD, others offer significantly different estimates:

> Hypothesis-driven studies on candidate genes ... are substantially influenced by the amount of existing knowledge regarding disease aetiology (sic). Since the knowledge of ADHD's cause is still limited ... such studies can explain

no more than 3–5% of the total genetic components of ADHD.[190] (Emphases are mine, as is this observation. We do not even have a 3-5% relationship between genes and ADHD. To do so, we'd need to know how to quantify the acronym, which would be like quantifying "love." On the other hand, we might discover a 3–5% relationship between genes *and* a child's *phenotype* since the child's behavior, at the data level, is quantifiable. Will we ever know the exact degree of that potential genetic relationship? Likely never. The nullifying environment begins its influence within hours of birth, if not before.)

Some children no doubt inherit tendencies toward the same or similar behavioral predispositions as their parents: talkative, reclusive, hasty, bookish, intense, easy-going, disorganized, impulsive, forgetful, obsessive, energetic—and with a motor that rarely shuts down. Genes, after all, are transmitted from generation to generation—though everyday behaviors (phenotypes) are introduced, and selectively strengthened, weakened, and continually modified by an early active environment that extends far beyond the family's influence. The selective differentiation may, in part, account for the following observations:

> Children in the same family are more similar than children taken at random from the population, but not much more. (Psychologist Robert Plomin) In terms of personality, we are similar to our siblings only about 20 percent of the time.[191]

Professional interests (may or may not) run in families. Doctor-parents produce doctor-children, except when they don't. Librarian-parents produce librarian-children who grow up to be librarian-parents. But librarian-parents also produce children of librarians who grow up banging away at drums in a traveling rock–and-roll band.

> [E]vidence supports what everyone's grandmother knew: there are inborn temperamental differences among children. Studies of the growth of children from infancy to preadolescence reveal that children differ from their earliest days and that some of these differences tend to be associated with behavioral problems as the child grows up.[192] In some families the children are high-strung (like fox terriers or cocker spaniels), whereas in others the children are more placid (like basset hounds). Any temperamental characteristic is not an all-or-none trait.[193]

How much of that dissimilarity is genetically or environmentally produced is the enduring nature/nurture question. The answer becomes more complicated the more we know, as we should expect.

> ...And our children's lives, with their mishmash of father's and mother's lineage, so much the more so. Even where children's genes look identical to their parents, their bodies and minds could well differ, influenced by many other factors, including the portions of the parents' DNA that don't code for genes, their environment, and their behavior. "Genetics is not destiny," said Dana Waring of the Personal Genetics Education Project, funded by a Harvard genetics lab. "The more we learn about genetics, the more complex and the more layered the story becomes."[194]

Any thinking person eagerly grants genes some ownership when considering how a child behaves at home and at school, some, but not to such a degree that we can't provide the child with more successful alternatives. That's as close genes come to ADHD-like behavior, the likelihood of influencing a child's temperament. Beyond that, ADHD, as a term that represents what kids do, isn't necessary.

The weak link in any genetic and/or neurobiological equation has always been ADHD. Without a reliable, valid ADHD diagnosis, no corroborating statement connecting ADHD with any causative factor can rightly be made either with regard to a child's genes or his/her neurology. As pointed out, you can't have a cause that yields an effect without having two variables, each of which satisfies the minimal prerequisites, being observable and measurable, both at the data level where there's something to see, validate, and agree upon. ADHD possesses none of those prerequisites. That limitation was certain to create problems for attribution studies.

> A major point that we would like to stress is that ... findings from genetic studies do not imply that genes are the only and exclusive factor in the etiology of ADHD. It is well known that heritability does not imply genetic determination. ... One of the crucial steps in genetics research of ADHD has been the acknowledgement of the interaction between genes and the environment. That environmental factors do play a significant role in the etiology of ADHD is unquestionable. One of the best evidence supporting this point comes from ... twin studies showing that the risk of ADHD in MZ twins [monozygotic twins] is much less than 100%.[195]

The statement "much less than 100%" tells us that *nongenetic* factors, some known, some unknown, contribute to the foundation of a child's ADHD-like *behaviors* (Box 4.5).

Box 4.5   ADHD

Cause	*Disorder*	*Behaviors*
Neurobiological, genetic factors non-genetic factors	ADHD	Counterproductive behaviors

Given the results geneticists have reported with regard to genes and ADHD, coupled with what we know about ADHD and the lack of any empirically supported neurological foundation, CHADD's chart needs modification. While the chart's adjusted form may appear meager, it's precisely where it needs to be. Nothing strategically is lost (Box 4.6).

Box 4.6   ADHD

Behaviors	*Cause*
Counterproductive behaviors	Unknown

Summary ADHD, as a medical or educational disorder, is neither observable nor measurable. Like pneumonia, like learning disabilities, ADHD has been from its inception a convenient shorthand acronym intended to make conversation easier. With respect to ADHD, we made that decision in the 1980s when we voted it into existence. Trying to *explain* a child's counterproductive behavior by suggesting the child has ADHD will remain a futile, tautological exercise. We do not diagnose created educational acronyms. Straw will remain straw no matter how long we spin it.

A CONFIRMABLE DISORDER

I'll provide you a reference point that will help you evaluate ADHD as a bona fide disorder, a prerequisite to any research, genetic-attribution or otherwise. If psychiatry's ADHD met the following criteria, arguments would cease to exist.

We're back in time, in the 1850s or thereabouts, in a remote English village in the UK. A rooster is about to crow, and a blessed event is about to take place.

Aided by a midwife, a female infant is born to Caucasian parents of European descent. Noticed immediately, the child possesses unusual physical qualities: low muscle tone, flat facial features, small nose, an upward slant to the eyes, small skin folds on the inner corner of the eyes, irregular shape of the tongue and mouth, and a single deep crease across the center of both palms where two relatively parallel lines were expected.

The facial characteristics stun the parents (and the midwife) as they compare the newborn with the family's other two children who stand close by. The peaceful infant with the unexpected features otherwise boasts a healthy skin color, normal breathing, golden hair, and rich dark chocolate eyes. The discordance is startling.

John Langdon Down

The mystery surrounding the child would fall to John Langdon Down, an English physician, who in 1866 published an accurate description of such infants. What caused the variation was unknown, and would remain so for nearly 100 years till a French physician, Jérôme Lejeune, with the advantage of a sophisticated microscope, noticed that the features occurred when an infant's genotype possessed 47 chromosomes rather than the predicted 46. It was later determined that the injurious extra chromosome was that of the 21st,[196] ultimately resulting in the genetic demarcation "trisomy 21." It would soon be recognized that in line with genetic laws, every child born with some configuration of the extra 21st chromosome would exhibit some or all of the features John Langdon Down described. Likewise, every Caucasian child of European descent born with the features John Langdon Down described would possess some configuration of an extra 21st chromosome.

The term "Down syndrome" is used to describe the presence of the 21st chromosome, the body tone and features, and many other physiological complications that often accompany the genetic variant, e.g., possible heart defects and thyroid disorders.

Our familiar chart referencing Down syndrome would look as follows (Box 4.7).

Box 4.7   Down syndrome

Symptoms	Convenient Construct	Cause
Physiological complications; physical features; cognitive, emotional, and behavioral irregularities	Down syndrome	Biologic/chemical contributions from a third 21st chromosome

Down syndrome's identification and verification fit comfortably within the medical model. The syndrome's current diagnostic process is accepted without opposition.

(FYI: Down syndrome is a convenient, universally accepted, shorthand construct. But like all constructs, the term "Down syndrome" fails to provide any indication of a child's social or intellectual strengths.)

Down syndrome's diagnostic sequence begins as it does with all established biological irregularities—with the observation of discrepant physical features, what ultimately become the symptoms that are associated with a biogenetic anomaly. In the case of *suspected* Down syndrome, once the physical symptoms had been identified, the facial features among those physical signs, attention would turn to verification *or* refutation of the predicted additional 21st chromosome. Exploration is accomplished by taking a snapshot—a photomicrograph of the child's chromosomes. If the additional third 21st chromosome were not verified, the name "Down syndrome" would *not* be used, and further diagnostic efforts to explain the child's unexpected differences would get under way.

This welcome diagnostic precision is made possible in part because the variables involved with Down syndrome are observable, measurable, confirmable, and on occasion refutable, prerequisites essential to all traditional diagnostic efforts. The resulting diagnosis is simple and straightforward. One hundred minimally trained people from all walks of life could verify and agree upon the presence of the physical features and the presence of the additional 21st chromosome. What's referred to as "inter-judge-" or "inter-rater reliability" is very high, meaning the observers (without conversing among themselves) see pretty much the same thing. (You've heard it said that ten people witnessing an automobile accident usually hold ten different perceptions of what transpired. That's *low* inter-judge reliability.)

Does a child *have* Down syndrome? "Down syndrome" is, after all, a shorthand construct. Therefore, technically, the child with the unusual facial features does *not* have Down syndrome, though no harm is done if the erred statement is made. (To be precise, the child *has* a genetic anomaly, a third 21st chromosome.) The erred statement that the child *has* Down syndrome is acceptable because Down's causal variable, the 21st chromosome, is established. It's well documented that the chromosomal abnormality has occurred as a random event during the formation of reproductive cells in a parent.[197] Once the genotype has been verified, we don't need to concern ourselves with a *second* (alternative) causal (or contributing) factor that rightly explains the *physical symptoms*.** [**See below, please.] Those symptoms *are* genetic in origin. The point as it relates to ADHD is most important and necessitates a quick word.

(FYI A: Down syndrome and the additional 21st chromosome are *interlocked* and exclusive to each other. Saying a child has Down syndrome is the same as saying the child has trisomy 21, and vice versa. But recall Sir Alexander Crichton's explanation for the children's fidgets—"fevered state of nerves." Squirming on one's bottom and fevered nerves are *not* interlocked and not at all exclusive. You can definitely have one without having the other—however one supposes to measure and thus verify Crichton's inventive "fevered nerves." With respect to the youngsters Crichton observed, the kids' fidgets were more likely the outcome of the teacher's curriculum that drove the youngsters bonkers. That hypothesis was testable; Crichton's "fevered nerves" was not.)

What happens if we fail to take into consideration a second possible explanation for observed behaviors when the etiology is uncertain or unknowable? We'll explain all children who fidget the same way, precisely Crichton's choice.

I'd like to say we're more progressive today, that prior to ADHD medication, we'd tweak a teacher's lesson and examine what effect, if any, the modification had on the children's behavior. In most cases, we don't. Sadly, many prescribing physicians follow Crichton's order of things. In fairness to the physician, the classroom teacher should have carried out the tweaking long before the medical doctor was contacted. That's an educational system problem, and a serious one.

**(FYI B: It's important to differentiate between physical symptoms associated with Down syndrome and social and educational behaviors that are often observed with the diagnosed children. The social and educational behaviors are not necessarily related to the child's genotype. The behaviors are often acquired in connection with how the environment responds to those behaviors, meaning that those behaviors are modifiable. The mistake easily made is to suggest that genes, by way of the syndrome, are responsible for a Down child's stubborn behavior or absence of focus or noncompliance. While the physical features may be interlocked, the child's behaviors are not. A good special education teacher and/or behavioral psychologist can devise effective programs to help the children acquire productive behaviors, the construct "Down syndrome" not relevant.)

In summary, we're determined to force ADHD into the medical model.

- We want to make ADHD more than a name.
- We want it to be an entity with a neurological and/or genetic foundation.
- We want to say that the social environment plays little role in the acquisition of ADHD-like behaviors that represent its supposed symptoms.
- We want to make ADHD a biological disorder to have.
- We want ADHD to be similar in kind to Down syndrome, with a verified biological base and a verified set of symptoms.
- We want to say that ADHD's diagnosis, like that of Down syndrome, is reliable, accurate and without controversy.
- We want to say that 100 minimally trained people would recognize ADHD with ease—we want the 100 people to believe that if they see children in a classroom who draw constant criticism from teachers they're witnessing children with ADHD.

Down syndrome is verifiable. ADHD is not. Down syndrome is diagnosable. ADHD, the proposed disorder, is not (see below, please). Down syndrome affords a replicable diagnostic methodology that every clinician can use reliably. ADHD does not. Drs. Moffitt and Melchior[198] can declare that Down syndrome is a bona fide disorder. They cannot validly say the same about ADHD.

DIAGNOSTICS

In place of asking what a child has, the essential diagnostic question must ask what a child *needs*.

The verb "diagnose" and the noun "diagnosis" are medical model terms. Like the model itself, they're well suited for the work carried out in hospitals and other medical facilities. To develop a diagnosis in the traditional sense of the term, the diagnostician must be seeking an observable, measurable entity, one with identifiable parameters with reliable, agreed upon form, shape, mass, weight, along with other possible signifiers. ADHD, the proposed disorder, lacks all of those essential features, yet because we've aligned ourselves with the medical model, we persist in speaking of the construct as if it is diagnosable. As you'll now see, we, at best, designate a child ADHD in order to provide the youngster accommodations and/or medication, what schools and medical ethics require. If you'll look closely at the following questionable methods, including the instruments we use in this identification process, you might wonder what it is that we're identifying.

> A child who shows five troubling symptoms [behaviors] as reported by a teacher *doesn't* meet [ADHD] criteria. A child needs six troubling symptoms [behaviors] to be diagnosed.[199] … [A] diagnostician is required to make an all-or-nothing decision. You count the symptoms. If [they] meet the criteria, then [the child is said to] "have" a psychiatric disorder.[200] If they don't, they don't. You've either got [ADD] or you don't.[201] (Emphasis mine)

> ADHD is controversial in part because most children are diagnosed and treated on the basis of data where the children's classroom teachers are the primary source of diagnostic information.[202] Remembering that "Teacher reports almost invariably come back as citing the behaviors that would warrant a diagnosis"[203] might give us pause.

A teacher standing in front of a class of children has little difficulty spotting behaviors that interfere with what he or she had planned for the group. In that position, s/he can decide if a behavior is disruptive enough to warrant intervention. It's rare that a physician or practicing psychologist has time to witness children in a classroom, or observe parents and their child at home, where the professional is intent on witnessing a child and the involved adult(s) interact in the context in which the interactions normally occur. Unless the professional chooses to spend countless hours (over a period of many days, perhaps weeks) observing a child under myriad conditions, the clinician must rely on information provided mostly by harried teachers (and hassled parents) who have observed, often haphazardly, a child's maddening behavior. How the clinician interprets the information relating to the child's behavior is dependent upon the clinician's training.

As we learned earlier when discussing Down syndrome, diagnosing the syndrome's variables is accomplished without difficulty or controversy. Diagnosing the variables associated with pneumonia is likewise well established and mostly free from subjectivity. Additionally, the signs and symptoms lend themselves to direct observation in a clinician's office, the time involved minimal. The stress on the physician to accurately diagnosis is virtually nonexistent.

ADHD, conversely, presents many problems.

> We're told that an accurate ADHD diagnosis can take two hours—or considerably more,[204] and that the process itself is only as good as the exceptional diagnostician.

A child's ADHD-like signs and behaviors, as varied as the children themselves, are seen briefly, if at all, by an office-bound physician or psychologist. Unlike the pneumonia-sufferer who brings with her the fever and cough, or the Down syndrome child who wears his physical features in plain view, a vexing youngster brought to see a physician or psychologist might present himself or herself as cooperative, interested, and pleasantly responsive throughout the total span of the physician's 15-minute visit. (Clinical psychologists are more inclined to abide by Robert Mitchell Lindner's 50-minute hour visit.)

> Perhaps the most damaging evidence of how vague the idea of ADD/ [ADHD] really is comes from studies that look at whether physicians can reliably diagnose children in their offices, the most common locations for diagnosis today. Because children who behave within the boundaries of acceptable behavior sometimes look hyperactive and because active children often look "normal," especially in the doctor's office, this poses a grave problem. One study, reported in the journal *Pediatrics,* found that 80 percent of the children thought to be hyperactive, according to home and school reports, showed "exemplary" behavior and no signs of hyperactivity in the office. This finding is consistent with numerous studies showing, and dozens of newspaper articles reporting, considerable disagreement among parents, teachers, and clinicians about who qualifies for an [ADHD] diagnosis.[205]

The astute physician and certainly a behaviorally trained psychologist, both inclined to believe a complaining teacher or parent, might acknowledge the quiet, compliant child knowing full well that the worrisome behaviors the youngster exhibits are often "stimulus-specific," meaning they don't occur all the time under all conditions. These "situational displays," as they might be considered, may either mean a great deal or very little to the clinician depending upon his or her training. Clinicians schooled in the ecological/behavioral model, rather than the medical model, know the importance of such stimulus-specific manifestations. The knowledgeable behaviorally trained clinician will provide parents of the well-behaved child with homework—requesting the folks run a diary to pinpoint what might prompt and/or contribute to the youngster's irksome behaviors. (Notice the absence of the term "cause.")

Not so clinicians vested entirely in biological pathology germane to the medical model. Given the quiet, cooperative child, the bemused clinician will know little else to do but wait for the hassled teacher or parent to repeat a visit or call in a day or three to request help, knowing already what the adult will say.

As alluded to, the data most physicians and psychologists use to make their ADHD diagnostic decisions derive in major part from scores obtained via rating scales, checklists, and questionnaires filled out by teachers and parents, instruments that assess an adult's perception of a child's behavior. Different perceptions among parents and teachers are a common occurrence, resulting in evaluations that may reflect the character and preferences of the evaluator more than that of the child being observed.

Teachers do not observe children neatly—as does a technician who eyes his subject through the lens of a dust-free microscope. Teachers, and parents as well, must focus on dozens of variables simultaneously while the current environment swirls around them. They must do more than count occurrences. They must interpret what they're observing, where often a child's momentary behavior is infused with ever-changing nuances. If a teacher's judgment is inaccurate, the inaccuracies will be recorded and relayed as such. The diagnostician in his or her office will assume the teacher/parent collected the data accurately when the opposite might be more likely. Diagnostic decisions made about a child, might be wrong, as might be the resulting treatment. Most troubling is that neither the parent, nor the teacher, nor the diagnostician may be aware of any observational and recording errors. Given that scores taken from questionnaires, checklists, and rating scales carry enormous diagnostic weight, their variability, subjectivity, and probable error raise the specter of diagnostic tools that are unreliable and invalid for the task assigned.

Medical model people believe ADHD is diagnosable. They believe they can make an accurate diagnosis. Their methods, what we will look at now, will verify if their confidence is justified. If their diagnostic methods are lacking, their assertions about ADHD will be reduced to pure speculation.

> Researchers created a double-blind ADHD study to test how much agreement there would be among people making assessments of children as "better, same, or worse." They compared ratings given by parents and by teachers, as well as by [non-classroom staff]. … They found no agreement among raters. In fact, raters were "more likely to disagree than agree."[206]

CONFIRMING ADHD

Three interrelated procedures are used to establish the coveted ADHD diagnosis:

- An assortment of questionnaires, checklists, and rating scales
- Psychiatry's own Diagnostic and Statistical Manual of Mental Disorders (DSM)
- A clinician's personal judgment

(FYI: The Diagnostic and Statistical Manual of Mental Disorders (DSM) is a reference book used by clinicians and researchers to diagnose and classify mental disorders. The manual is published by the American Psychiatric Association and covers all mental health disorders for both children and adults. In the case of ADHD, the DSM lists the behaviors clinicians use to build a diagnosis. In addition, the DSM sets out for the clinician the conditions a child must meet in order to be diagnosed with ADHD. Most important, the child must exhibit a minimum number of ADHD-like behaviors under varying conditions to meet criteria. The DSM is the most relied upon source to establish an ADHD diagnoses. The manual is not without controversy. [See below, please.])

The first two diagnostic methods (questionnaires etc. and the DSM's list of behaviors and qualifiers) serve as a physician's stethoscope, though almost exclusively measured through the eyes and ears of *others*. The third, clinical judgment, interprets a breadth of information, often including what's provided by the two approaches. The three diagnostic approaches are not separate and equal, however. A weakness in any one of the three will result in conflicting and thus confusing information that's bound to impact a clinician's judgment. (I've included a fourth diagnostic method. It's presented for its interest, not its utility.)

All three approaches collectively measure and evaluate an adult's recollection and judgment as they pertain to a child's behavior. Though the evaluated child's behavior never occurs in isolation, it's safe to suggest that none of the analyses take into account the functional influences the child's environment has had on the behavior being judged. The medical model assumes that a child's ADHD behaviors are driven exclusively by the child's biology. It believes the child's environment plays no major role, placing it at odds with the points made by Drs. Hinshaw and Scheffler who concurred that the child's parents, as well as others in the child's environment, do impact what a child does. If it can be shown that a child's behavior is to a large extent influenced by what s/he experiences, then the youngster's behavior, rather than being disordered, would be adaptive to the lessons the evironment has been teaching. That would not be ADHD.

Evaluators observe and record the frequencies of the child's troubling behavior, though their estimates are certain to be inexact. The evaluator reports those frequencies to the clinician, who has little option but to conclude a one-to-one relationship between what's recorded and what is accurate. The clinician counts the symptoms reported and decides what the numbers mean. The DSM makes the professional decision fairly simple.

> You count the symptoms [the child's behaviors.] If [they] meet the criteria, then [the child is said to] "have" a psychiatric disorder.[207]

The clinician may conclude with or without confidence that the child *has* ADHD. If asked to support the contention, the physician or psychologist will most likely point at the child's behaviors as described by the evaluators. Chances are the clinician will be unaware that his or her judgment is tautological, and the conclusion that the child has ADHD is unconfirmable. The diagnostic method is what's at fault.

The Pivotal Flaw

Before we examine the three data collection methods traditional clinicians use to make their ADHD diagnosis, it's necessary to understand the basic principle that underlies all ADHD diagnostic decisions, a principle summed up accurately when psychologist Tom Brown asked,

> To whom should an individual be compared with to make a diagnosis of ADHD?[208]

In his book, *Attention Deficit Disorder*, Dr. Brown mentioned that sometimes a teacher feels strongly that a child has an ADHD-impairment while neither parent sees such a problem. Or parents may see ADHD indicators in their child's efforts to do homework...and social relationships, while the child's teacher reports no evidence of any such difficulties at school, confirming once again the variability of the behaviors associated with ADHD as well as adult evaluators' judgments.

More enlightening, Dr. Brown reports that two researchers found that although parents and teachers disagreed considerably on the number of symptoms a child had, they more often agreed about whether the child was impaired *relative to others*.[209] "Relative to others" speaks directly to Tom Brown's opening question: To whom should an individual be compared to make a diagnosis of ADHD?

Diagnosticians working to develop a diagnosis of ADHD often make their diagnostic decision only after judging a child against other children of similar age. Recall the earlier case where the child whose parents were French was diagnosed almost exclusively with that mindset. After viewing a tape of the boy in his classroom, the psychologist concluded, "It was pretty apparent that he was below average in his ability to just stay in one place." That's a normative comparison. The child's actual behavior was less important than how that behavior compared to others. The presumption: if all the children in the class were equally derelict in their ability to stay in one place, ADHD would not be offered as an explanation. Such comparisons may occur subliminally, or they may be blatant. I knew a social worker who diagnosed children as "emotionally disturbed" only after comparing them to her own children. A convenient, if not a questionable, approach. Interview teachers who work in a crowded classroom and you'll see the same approach. A teacher will point to a disruptive child and contrast him/her with those youngsters seated nearby. If that teacher fills out forms used to assess ADHD, that comparative incident will influence how she scores the child, and eventually how the clinician diagnoses the child.

Tom Brown's reference "relative to others" exposes a weakness in ADHD's diagnostic scheme, specifically the need to compare one child against others to determine if one or the other is disordered. ADHD is not determined based on its own perceived pathology, as would be the case with pneumonia presenting its respiratory symptoms, or measles, with its fever, sore throat, and Koplik spots. With Dr. Brown's "To whom should an individual be compared with...," ADHD becomes "normative" where a child is disordered based on a head count, again reflective of the psychologist who evaluated the French boy. The logic appears to be that if most children do something, the behavior must be normal. The converse, of course, follows suit. If a child doesn't do what most do, the child is at greater risk of being diagnosed disordered.

By comparing kids, the designation ADHD isn't child-dependent but rather child-*interdependent*. Prior to suggesting a child has ADHD, s/he must be matched to either the mythical average-aged child or a presumed acceptable developmental level based on age and majority. That's head count again.

There's a major problem with the comparative approach. To be valid, comparisons between the child and the chosen standard require that the children's environments have had no differential influence on the children's behavior, otherwise the environments, in addition to the child's biology, become shared factors affecting what any given child does. Put differently, for the "head-count" to be acceptable, all children of the same age must be influenced in the exact same way by their everyday environmental experiences. If the environment influences the children differentially, then the children's behaviors are less driven by any hypothesized gene or neurological base, and more by their environmental experiences, weakening an ADHD hypothesis.

Unlike childhood ailments such as mumps, chickenpox, strep, and the like, where a child is obviously suffering from a compromised biology, ADHD, the disorder, needs a crowd to exist. Change the group of children with whom a target child is compared, and the child may appear less impulsive, less inattentive, less hyperactive—even though his or her behavior has remained the same. Place a quiet, solitary achiever in a self-aggrandized, powerhouse of a school where every child, for the sake of the school's reputation, is pushed to excel, and the private, quiet, self-sufficient child is likely to draw the kind of attention that attaches itself to ADHD. Move the same child to a school where humble, steady achievement is appreciated and supported, and the purported disorder will no longer be part of the child's life space. Has the child changed? No. His surroundings have.

Nearly 1 million children in the U.S. have been misdiagnosed because of what the authors called, "relative age effect." The relative age effect states that the youngest children in a classroom are frequently misdiagnosed as having ADHD when more likely their increased active behaviors are explained by the fact that they are at a different developmental stage than their older classmates.[210]

Specifically:

> Kindergarten children who were the youngest for their grade—late 4 or early 5—had a 60% higher chance of receiving an ADHD diagnosis and medication than those entering in the middle of the age cluster.[211] A 2010 study carried out in Canada suggested that younger boys were 39% more likely to be diagnosed ADHD than their slightly older counterparts. The misdiagnosis percentage was even greater with girls.[212]

If our topic were penguins residing in Antarctica or the Galápagos, we could successfully determine appropriate and inappropriate symptoms/ behavior based exclusively on developmental age. The engaging creatures *are* preprogrammed to proceed through a linear developmental sequence that's related to the passing of time and the rising and setting of the sun, the environment, with little impact other than, perhaps, to have helped teach the little guys to huddle close during a winter blizzard (though that adaptive behavior might be DNA-coded as well). But comparing human kids is infinitely more complicated—and, excluding exceptions like first-word, first-step milestones, a decidedly poor choice to make. That the medical model mandates as a diagnostic marker that the child's behavior "must be inappropriate for the child's developmental age"[213] reveals its authors' bizarre thinking that all kids run on internal Timex clocks, and differences among the kids are signs of malfunctioning lithium batteries. You'd think these professionals had never heard of gene variations and environmental influences, factors that in the end produce each child as a unique self.

The concept of "developmentally inappropriate", again, says that all six years, by the fact that they are six, should have developed at the same speed, and all should be manifesting the same behavior, its frequency, its topography, its intensity. After comparing the children, the one whose behavior is developmentally *different* and thus *inappropriate* is often designated disordered. The conclusion requires that the clinician discounts any environmentally produced learning that may have contributed to the child's differences. Acknowledging that the environment might play a role in the child's differences challenges ADHD's biological roots.

RATING BEHAVIORS

The official ADHD diagnostic sequence usually starts with our often discussed checklists, questionnaires, or rating scales.[214] These devices ask parents and teachers to determine the frequency of bothersome behaviors.

Those behaviors are most often derived from the list of behaviors found in the DSM. (See below, please.) These checklists, questionnaires, and rating scales and their produced numbers determine in large measure whether a diagnosis of ADHD is made.

Clinicians who use questionnaire data to help them make decisions must

- Assume the reliability of the instruments being used to assess the child
- Assume the reliability of the individuals administering and scoring the instrument
- Predict that a dozen different teachers/parents viewing the same child would score that youngster in identical fashion
- Assume truth in numbers—*in numeris veritas*: that the collected and reported numbers are real, and that the score truly represents that child's behavior. Teacher/parent ratings provide a clinician checkmarks that represents the number of symptoms observed. The clinician knows to count the checkmarks. The symptoms observed and counted aren't as precise as body temperature.[215]

Assessment of a child's behavior is hampered by the vagueness of the descriptive choices evaluators are forced to make. Consider that a teacher or parent decides that a disturbing child "often does not seem to listen when spoken to directly." That exact behavior is an ADHD-like symptom listed in the fifth (and latest) revision of the DSM. To facilitate the rating process, the evaluator is provided a scale to use to assess the frequency of the "not-listening" behavior. As is apparent, the DSM's designation "often" requires that the evaluator decide how often is often. Once a week could be too much for one teacher, while another might tolerate multiple repetitions before considering the behavior worrisome. That variability is a factor that introduces possible (and unknown) error into the diagnostic equation.

The evaluator's emotional disposition further challenges the assessment procedure. Prior to rating, the parent or teacher who's judging the child may not be in the most objective of moods, given the real possibility that the youngster may have been doing to the adult what a jet-powered blender does to an egg white. It's only after the adult is thoroughly annoyed with a child's behavior that s/he seeks an ADHD diagnosis. It's not as if the adult is anxious over a child's fever or facial flushness or uncharacteristic weariness. The adult, more often than not, is harried and besieged, not worried. Still, the adult is required to objectively estimate the behavior's frequency. S/he must choose from the following available answers, several as difficult to grasp as a withering cloud.

- "Yes" or "No," or "not true at all," "just a little true," "pretty much true," or "very much true."[216]
- One scale's ratings include "never," "occasionally," "often," "very often," while another adds to the these selections "almost always."
- One provided "just a little," and "quite a bit."
- Some scales ask evaluators to rate by numbers 1–5, where 1 is never and 5 is several times an hour.

Suppose our evaluator were an overextended teacher with 30 assigned children and no assistant. Suppose she's determined to obtain a diagnosis of ADHD—and the medication that frequently comes with it, hoping at least to regulate pharmaceutically one of several energetic, less academically motivated pupils. She reads the behavior reference, which states that this is a child "who often does not seem to listen when spoken to directly." The teacher must decide how the statement reflects upon the *energetic, unmotivated, bothersome* child. "Pretty much true," she marks without much thinking, remembering the tussle she had with him earlier in the day, having to remind him three times to find his seat and stop talking to friends. Her rating might reflect her personal agenda rather than an accurate estimate.

> The ADHD diagnostic scoring process has been described as "pretty low-tech,"[217] hardly the stuff that elicits the same confidence as counting a patient's red blood cells.

What does the designation "pretty much true" really mean? What some teachers (and stressed parents), in their haste to find some relief, might overlook. Pretty much true means the child who doesn't listen...*does* listen. It's a start, and an important one. The same if the teacher had scored, "Often doesn't," "occasionally doesn't," "almost always doesn't," even "very much true...doesn't."

(FYI: If we're in this business to do more than label/diagnose a child disordered, "pretty much" says that sometimes the child does precisely what the teacher (or parent) wants him/her to do. That could be (should be) cause for celebration, particularly if we have a teacher who's interested in helping the youngster do better. "Pretty much true" means there are specific times during the day when the child does listen when spoken to directly. Always at certain times? Never at certain times? Give that information to a behaviorally trained psychologist or special education teacher and the idea of ADHD rapidly dissipates in favor of building on the desired behavior.)

Are ADHD-like children this variable? Are their behaviors so changeable? It seems logical that if a child *has* ADHD at 9:00 a.m, he or she will *have* ADHD at 11:00 and at 2:00. After all, if a child has a bad cold at 9:00, it's pretty much true that it's an all-day affair. Not so, an ADHD advocate advises:

> All the primary symptoms of ADHD show significant fluctuations across settings and caregivers.[218]

Why might a child do better at sometimes during a day, and do better with some people more than others? It's an important question. Something's going on that the child enjoys and appreciates. It would be helpful to know what it is, don't you think?

Without further information, options such as "almost always" and "pretty much true" are loose standards for making a diagnosis that may change a child's brain chemistry. Likewise (and more important for the child), such subjective estimates are of *no* help to a teacher who wishes to do more than label a youngster with the construct ADHD—or to any physician who is determined to do more than imprint a child officially disordered and provide medication. Yet if "pretty much" or "often" or "sometimes" is checked by the teacher who has several energetic youngsters, the child needs only a few more implicating ratings to meet ADHD criteria and be viewed as disordered—with no accompanying information that tells a teacher what's a first step toward a workable, successful strategy. It's a return to the ineffectual "naming game" where we believe that if we could just decide on a suitable name for a disorder we'd know what to do—beyond medicate. There's no truth to that belief. Additional problems plague these assessment tools that have acquired such diagnostic power and influence in deciding whether a school *child's* life will be changed. Chief among them: they attempt to measure activities, such as inattention and hyperactivity, that represent part of the normal spectrum of behavior. Because the symptoms of ADD occur in most children to some extent, it is only when there are enough of them in combination, when the child finally upsets his or her [parent or teacher], that a diagnosis [of ADHD] is deemed warranted. In short, the diagnosis is based on a vague system of counting the frequency of what would otherwise be considered normal behaviors.[219]

> Researchers reviewed several studies that asked teachers and parents to examine similar data regarding ADHD and various issues that were involved. In one study, parents and teachers were asked to estimate the genetic influence on children's attention difficulties. The parents and teachers were presented the same data. They differed markedly in their assessment, teachers estimating the influence at 39%, parents at 69%. When asked to estimate common genetic factors involving ADHD, teachers estimated 33%, parents 86%. The studies' authors suggested that the findings are indicative of rater effects, which can confound estimates. They concluded there were major problems involving variations of ratings.[220]

Supporters of these paper/pencil evaluation systems (and the DSM) are quick to point out that "It's not the behavior per se [that's important] but [the behavior's] frequency, intensity, and degree of impairment that *tip the scales.*" (Emphases are mine.)[221] I think the above statement means that we're expected to endure the child's bothersome behavior until we're about to scream. That doesn't sound like a healthy choice for the child or the parent or teacher.

Focusing on an ADHD diagnosis often results in unnecessary delays in providing services to all parties involved. While the diagnostic wheels turn, the child's bothersome behaviors become more entrenched. And as you may recall, with ADHD, you either (officially) got it or you don't got it, depending on the child's behavior count. If a clinician is from the "got it/ don't got" side of the street, and the child doesn't quite got it, the stickler for such details might advise the (abandoned) teacher, "Bring the kid back when things get worse," meaning when the behavior count is higher and the situation is more agonizing.

(FYI: Well-trained behavioral practitioners, especially school psychologists and special education teachers don't wait for the scales to tip before assisting the youngster. Experience has taught them that when the scales finally do tip, the ship and its crew are half under water.)

Where did this attitude come from where we're to wait until the chaos reaches unbearable proportions before we intervene? General education staff saw this "pretty-much-not-listening" child a mile back. Why didn't the educators intervene? Why didn't they help the child learn to listen more effectively? Here's why. Many of the public-school staff's administrators and general education teachers were taught in their college classes that the child's *problem* was a disorder called ADHD. They were taught ...

- ...that ADHD was a **medical** problem, that its cause was neurological and/or genetic,
- ...that a child's not listening had nothing to do with school or home or a life without structure or limits or redirection or incentives to do better,
- ...that the child's not listening had nothing to do with them or their parents, and
- most disconcertingly, that there was nothing they could do to help the child—and nothing the child could do to help himself or herself, that his behavior was ruled by his genes and/or his neurology.

They were taught *wrong*, the neuromyth[222] firmly planted.

In summary, questionnaires, checklists, and rating scales sample crudely an adult's subjective, unconfirmed perception of a child's behavior as designated by vague descriptors that provide limited information. Under pressure to arrive at a diagnosis, these vague approximations that are derived from the smallest representative sample of a child's behavior, with values that mean very little, are transformed into finite numbers that are interpreted to mean a lot. That's a shell game. Shaky grounds upon which to make important decisions about someone else's child. Making diagnostic decisions on the basis of these instruments represents the need for expediency at the expense of good science. If these instruments are the basis of an ADHD diagnosis, that diagnosis is highly suspect.

> A score on the Conners Teacher Rating Scale, or any of the other scales used in (an ADHD) diagnosis, gives the appearance of scientific precision, as though it were, say, a white-cell count. In reality, the score is nothing more than a numerical value that sums up a particular teacher's subjective judgments about whether a child bounces around too much.[223]

THE DSM

The concept of ADHD was developed to rationalize a preexisting motivation with medicine and psychology to use stimulant drugs to control the behavior of children. From the beginning, the focus was on classroom settings in which one-to-one attention is not available. ADHD as a diagnosis evolved as a convenient list of various behaviors that tend to disrupt a classroom and to require additional or special attention from teachers or other adults. Almost every behavior that tries a teacher's ability or patience, or drains a teacher's energy and attention, has been put into the diagnosis.[224,225]

CHADD Speaker: "Attention Deficit Disorder is a hidden disability. No physical marker exists to identify its presence, yet ADD/[ADHD] is not very hard to spot. Just look with your eyes and listen with your ears when you walk through places where children are—particularly those places where children are expected to behave in a quiet, orderly, and productive fashion. In such places, children...will identify themselves quite readily. They will be doing or not doing something which frequently results in their receiving a barrage of comments and criticisms such as 'Why don't you ever listen?' 'Think before you act.' 'Pay attention.'"[226]

"...[M]y own work with these [ADHD] children suggests that noncompliance is also a primary problem."[227] —Russell Barkley, PhD

The conjectured causes associated with ADD/ADHD, "from brain damage...to dysfunctional families [have] never been confirmed by research," leaving the diagnostician the remaining option to "retreat to a position of simply describing the symptoms."[228] "We are left with a disorder whose diagnosis is based solely on symptoms,"[229] where "the symptoms [the child's behaviors] are the disease."[230] In other words, "Despite 'strenuous efforts at standardization,' diagnosis [of ADHD] is best characterized as 'in-the-eye-of-the-beholder.'"[231]

Please understand the importance of Box 4.8.

Box 4.8   ADHD

A Child's Behaviors

It's what we have.

The following represents the DSM's list of ADHD-like behaviors. They're divided between "attention behaviors" and behaviors suggestive of "hyperactivity and impulsivity." Pragmatically, the child's behaviors and what drives them are all that matter, even more than the name ADHD. Ask a stressed teacher or distraught parent if they agree with that statement and each will confirm that the name is secondary to helping the child behave differently. Recall, please, that a well-behaved, compliant, responsible child is never diagnosed ADHD. Recall, too, that we must teach a child to be well-behaved and compliant.

Inattention:
The child

- Often fails to give close attention to details or makes careless mistakes in schoolwork, at work, or with other activities
- Often has trouble holding attention on tasks or play activities
- **Often does not seem to listen when spoken to directly**
- Often does not follow through on instructions and fails to finish schoolwork, chores, or duties in the workplace (e.g., loses focus, side-tracked)
- Often has trouble organizing tasks and activities
- Often avoids, dislikes, or is reluctant to do tasks that require mental effort over a long period of time (such as schoolwork or homework)
- Often loses things necessary for tasks and activities (e.g., school materials, pencils, books, tools, wallets, keys, paperwork, eyeglasses, mobile telephones)
- Is often easily distracted
- Is often forgetful in daily activities

Hyperactivity and Impulsivity: Behaviors
The child

- Often fidgets with or taps hands or feet, or squirms in seat
- Often leaves seat in situations when remaining seated is expected
- Often runs about or climbs in situations where it is not appropriate (adolescents or adults may be limited to feeling restless)
- Often unable to play or take part in leisure activities quietly
- Often "on the go" acting as if "driven by a motor"
- Often talks excessively
- Often blurts out an answer before a question has been completed
- Often has trouble waiting his/her turn

- Often interrupts or intrudes on others (e.g., butts into conversations or games)

Questionnaires, rating scales, and checklists are built substantially on the DSM's list of "inattention" and "hyperactivity" behaviors. According to the DSM, the behaviors exhibited by a child represent symptoms of ADHD, where ADHD is the driving force behind the behaviors.

(FYI: ADHD is not the driving force, not the answer to the perplexing question that seeks to learn what specifically produces a child's disturbing behavior. The best answer? Genes, in part, certainly, neurology, in part, certainly, though their specifics are unconfirmed. The environment, certainly, but how much is unknown, if unknowable. The etiological puzzle that explains a child's troublesome behavior is, as suggested early on, not easily solved.)

If a child is observed to exhibit 6 of the above behaviors over time and under different circumstances, the youngster can be said to have a psychiatric disorder. What appears neat and tidy is not. The DSM's diagnostic cutoffs represent a major problem.

If we were counting white blood cells, or diagnosing Type 2 diabetes, we'd have valid and reliable cutoff scores that would alert physicians to the existence of a serious discrepancy. Medical science knows when blood levels and cell counts are demanding immediate intervention.

But ADHD has nothing in common with cells and blood levels. We're counting occasional behaviors a child's exhibits,

- Behaviors that are in great measure learned.
- Behaviors that are often culturally bound.
- Behaviors whose frequency is continuously increased and decreased by teacher and parent reactions, not by a child's biology.

(FYI: If, as psychologist Barkley suggested, that noncompliance is a primary problem for ADHD-kids, it's because the children haven't been taught to be compliant. Teach the kids compliance and they become less ADHD-like. Non-compliance's absence doesn't call into question the children's biology, but their teachers'/parents' skills.)

Psychiatry tried to emulate laboratory precision. They stipulated that five or fewer behavioral issues would not constitute ADHD, whereas six or more marked behaviors would permit a diagnosis of ADHD and allow a physician to prescribe drugs. (That's the got it/don't got it mentality.) Devising behavioral cutoffs where at or above a particular count is pathological, and near and below are within acceptable limits, is about as foolish (and non-functional) as stipulating that sustained winds at 74 mph constitute a hurricane, whereas sustained winds at 73 mph do not. Does a homeowner decide to protect or not protect windows on the basis of that one mph?

Consider a child's disruptive behaviors at home or in the classroom, disturbing behaviors that the child discovered gained him/her access to what s/he wanted. It happens, and the behavior is adaptive and its learned and someone had to teach the lesson. Is 6 of those acquired behaviors that much more disconcerting than 5? Is 5 that much less upsetting than 6? With 5, does the parent or teacher have to wait until life gets more unbearable to receive help? Aware of the capricious cutoff, and with only five symptom/behaviors documented, is the desperate parent or teacher not primed to manufacture a sixth?

(FYI: A thoughtful clinician, with less concern toward diagnosis and the ADHD label, would dismiss the illogical cutoff and suggest 5 disturbing behaviors were as debilitating as 6. More so, the same clinician, if behaviorally trained, and cognizant of prevention, would suggest that even 1 problem behavior observed in school or home would warrant some discussion if not an immediate intervention.)

If whimsical diagnostic cutoffs weren't enough to raise serious questions about the DSM's diagnostic procedure's authenticity, the collection of the data a clinician uses to make a decision adds more than enough to raise serious questions. Reports parents and teachers provide a physician are confounded by several interrelated variables:

- The DSM language associated with ADHD is general and vague.[232]
- The behaviors children exhibit that professionals use in the diagnostic process are difficult to distinguish from everyday problems altogether unrelated to any proposed disorder.[233]
- The heightened tension and emotions of the evaluating adults that assure personal interpretation can result in embellishment if not exaggeration. These biases are seldom taken into account,"[234] biases that can produce over- and under-estimates of the behavior the child exhibits.

The DSM's non-operationalized list of behaviors that comprise the questionnaires and checklists used by teachers and parents are certain to result in conflicting evaluations. Two evaluators observing the same child and the same behavior might see both the child and what s/he's doing differently. That inconsistency is a serious problem that threatens the validity of the entire diagnostic process, as are the following failings:

- The evaluators aren't always objective observers.
- The evaluators have scant records that might illuminate the behaviors' lengthy or abbreviated history.
- The evaluators' observations are often one-shot carried out under pressured time constraints.
- The majority of the questionnaire and checklist answer-options are nebulous to the point of distraction where flipping a coin affects the decision.
- The cutoff scores that ultimately result in a diagnosis are arbitrary and without any science behind them.
- The data provided the clinician never consider the child within the context of his or her complex life where the psychologist or physician might gain a broader, more representative picture of the youngster. The clinician might choose to assist the parent or teacher rather than considering medication for the child.

Then there's an additional issue that compromises the DSM's diagnostic process, one that supersedes all the others, one that medical model proponents often fail to consider.

Even if the evaluators were well trained and unaffected by personal agendas, even if the questionnaires were reliable, and the numbers collected represented accurate accounts of a child's in-class or in-home behaviors, even if the DSM's markers were operationalized at the data language level, even *then* not listening, not focusing, not concentrating, making careless mistakes on tests, losing school materials, even getting up out of a chair while all the other students sit patiently, would still *not* be signs of an ADHD-disordered brain. Suggesting otherwise is the *medicalization* of the child.

Children can *choose* to listen or choose not to listen. They can choose to follow or not follow directions. Listening is volitional, and thus optional. A child's genes or his/her neurology do *not* drive the youngster's listening. Unlike gaining a tooth that is set in place by a developmental clock, listening is a voluntary behavior, under the control of an individual, with environmental influence, if a teacher or parent chooses to influence. Medical model people might disagree, declaring that teacher/parental influence is irrelevant, that the child doesn't listen, doesn't focus, because s/he can't listen and s/he can't focus, that his/her brain's wiring interferes. Likewise, the medical model people will opine that child can't sit, can't complete assignments, can't refrain from blurting, and can't remember what she did with her homework assignment, though she can remember the ice cream in the freezer. It is their mantra. To acknowledge that the child has a choice to do what diagnosticians suggest is biologically driven usurps ADHD as the *cause* of the child's counterproductive behavior. Choice means the child can weigh the pros and cons that are integral to the behavior. That's not ADHD.

The child's environment is a potent force, and many environmental factors impact a child's decision to listen, including a child's upbringing, prior success with answering questions, the moment's topic, the language (content and level) used, and whatever lessons the child has learned from family and friends how to behave in school. If a child fails to listen to a teacher's direction, even always, there exists a history behind the child's choice, a history not necessarily experienced by any other student in the class.

Is "not listening" to a teacher a desirable behavior? Not likely. But that doesn't qualify the behavior as a component of ADHD, which, I remind you, is not considered a proven disorder by everyone.[235]

The same can be said for most, if not all, of the DSM's other symptoms/behaviors under the category of inattention. They're learned, they're practiced, and they produce environmental consequences that affect their future occurrence. Again, they are voluntary actions children can choose to do or choose not to do. Whether the children participate depends in large measure on what they've been taught by a parent or a teacher. In school, a child may not do what is expected if s/he sees no reason to do what is expected. That's not pathological. That's adaptive. A poor choice, perhaps, but that's a separate issue. ADHD, even used as a descriptive label, excuses everyone and everything that currently influences the child. That's education's medical model, and it's altogether misplaced.

The DSM is the vehicle used to provide the child with a diagnosis. The diagnosis is the vehicle used most often to provide the child with medication. The child's active environment, what represents the life space within which the child lives, is removed from the process. We're determined to change the child almost exclusively through the use of ADHD-medication. In doing so we leave the environment as it is, both at home and at school, with no thought given to any adjustments. Some clinicians are satisfied with the outcome.

Estimates suggest that upwards to 70–80% of stimulant medicated children will behave somewhat better and may even be somewhat more productive in school. There is a secondary problem with that, however. It needs to be remembered that the pharmaceutical intervention is passive. It requires nothing from the child or the child's parents or teachers. In the process, the child learns nothing that would help him/her acquire self-directed behavior, which at some point in his/her life will be required.

In all of this, the DSM is irrelevant. The vehicle can have four flat tires and it still runs. It doesn't need to pass anyone's inspection. It gets lots of people where they want to go. That's enough for most to look at the end without seeing anything in between.

THE DSM'S GRADE: "F"

Physical medicine's accomplishments today are astounding. Today, medicine can peer into the soul of the smallest cell, understand many of its structures, tame some of its wildness, and provide for most cooperative people good health and long life. But the medical model often flounders *outside* its comfortable organic arena, in the school classroom, for example, where such terms as "symptom," "diagnosis," and "treatment" are borrowed and forced and are noticeably out of place:

- Where telltale discrepancies indeed exist, but the variables are social and curricular and are not biological.
- Where the concept of pathology doesn't fit any more than does the concept of normalcy as it pertains to groups of children.
- Where a child must be viewed within the context of his life, and not simply a product of disordered physiology.
- Where diagnosis should be ecological and not cellular.
- Where professionals understand there's no microscope through which to examine a school child's counterproductive behavior, that the specific behavior, to be understood and modified, must be viewed through the prism of a child's life that displays the youngster as the unique, adaptive individual he or she is.

The DSM's symptom count is conspicuously out of place. Diagnoses by way of symptom count mandate that we have some standard upon which to make a valid decision. The DSM professes to provide that standard. We assume, of course, that the measuring instrument provides a valid and reliable read. If not, then we have no valid diagnosis.

If, for example, our child complained of not feeling well, we might take her temperature. Noticing the reading of 103.4, we'd reflexively feel her forehead. If it felt cool, we might wonder about the thermometer. We'd check our own temperature with the same thermometer. If the instrument reads 103.4, we'd fetch little sister who was enjoying a bowl of ice cream. If her reading was also 103.4, we'd confidently assume that the measuring instrument was faulty. Faulty instruments result in faulty interpretations. The DSM as a diagnostic tool is, according to its credentialed critics, faulty.

STANDARDS

We've already discussed the weakness of diagnoses made when children are compared with one another in the absence of confirmed criteria. Personal biases influence subjective decisions and, in the final analysis, we're not certain if what we have (or have been told) is correct. A different set of problems surface when we diagnosis ADHD by comparing a child's behavior against a standard, where we diagnose a disorder by suggesting a child's impulsivity, inattention, and/or hyperactivity "is developmentally [age] inappropriate."[236]

Standards or norms (that are said to be developmental markers) require many thousands of random children, over multiple years, all who have demonstrated a specific behavior, e.g., sitting independently, the appearance of a first tooth, speaking a first word, taking a first step, each at an approximate point in time. Having passed that test, these standards, few as they are, legitimately become a respected measure against which behaviors are assessed, children are compared, and diagnoses are made. Any discussion of these standards or norms as they pertain to ADHD and the DSM's behaviors requires the mention of three important factors. First, normed behaviors must be well-defined, observable, and reliably measurable. A first tooth is a first tooth, not *pretty much* a first tooth. Our previously mentioned team of 100 observers, with little professional training, would agree that the object that has recently emerged through a baby's gums is a tooth. Correctness and accuracy are important when using standards and norms to make judgments. Second, even established standards/norms come with measured (and expected) time fluctuations, often sizable ranges. The appearance of first words can vary by many months, as can a baby's first step where the average first step occurs at roughly 13 months, while the range of average can extend from 10 to 16 months. Third, professionals do use standards to evaluate a child's development. Milestones are expected at approximate ages. An absence of the behaviors serves as a sign to be vigilant. Failure of a behavior to appear well after its expected time frame is reason to seek answers to important questions. Norms involving developmental behaviors are, therefore, very important aids.

"Listening," however, has *no* developmental norm or standard. Nor do *any* of the behaviors listed by psychiatry's DSM. Often, ADHD decisions made by physicians are based upon a teacher's or parent's level of frustration or anger elicited by a child's behavior, the DSM standard, subjective at best, providing the vehicle with which to make the diagnosis. Six named behaviors produce that diagnosis, the foundation with little to no objective, accountable science behind it. Overall, the DSM has received a failing grade.

> The often-heralded DSM represents an unscientific and subjective system of evaluation and classification. We're told that there exists "ongoing issues concerning the validity and reliability of the diagnostic categories; the reliance on superficial symptoms; the use of artificial dividing lines between categories; arbitrary cut-offs between normal and abnormal behavior; the possible presence of cultural bias, as well as the unwarranted medicalization of human distress."[237,238]

> Fads in psychiatric diagnosis come and go and have been with us as long as there has been a psychiatry. The fads meet a deeply felt need to explain, or at least to label, what would otherwise be unexplainable human suffering and deviance. In recent years the pace has picked up and false "epidemics" have come in bunches involving an ever-increasing proportion of the population. We are now in the midst of at least three such epidemics, [one of which is] attention deficit. ... Fads punctuate what has become a basic background of overdiagnosis. Normality is an endangered species. It is no accident that the recent "epidemics" have all occurred in the childhood disorders. There are two contributing factors. The first is the push by drug companies into this new market. The second is that the provision of special educational services often requires that there be a DSM diagnosis.[239]

The publication of the DSM, with tightly guarded copyrights, now returns to the American Psychiatric Association's coffers over 5 million a year, historically totaling over 100 million.[240] That might constitute a miracle of sorts if one examined the DSM closely enough to see its many flaws—and its propensity for overdiagnosis and overmedication. Although the DSM is often referred to as "psychiatry's bible,"—though it is "not [the] sacred scripture to all clinicians."[241]

DSM's effort at being diagnostically objective has been quite subjective. The way the DSM-IV committee chose criteria needed for a confirmed ADHD diagnosis was characterized as "arbitrary," their action having "little to do with science."[242] "Inner circle doubts" were raised years ago against the diagnostic procedure's validity and reliability.

> Today's classification of the major psychiatric disorders is as confusing as it used to be thirty years ago. All things considered, the present situation is worse. Then, psychiatrists were at least aware that diagnostic chaos reigned and many of them had no high opinions of diagnosis anyhow. Now, the chaos is codified and much more hidden.[243] (Dr. Herman van Pragg, former Head of the Department of Psychiatry at Albert Einstein College of Medicine)

Summarizing, "The [current] DSM-5 relies exclusively on fallible subjective judgments rather than objective biological tests. … It introduced several high-prevalence diagnoses at the fuzzy boundary with normality— one in particular, the already overused diagnosis of attention-deficit disorder. … Thanks to criteria that have been loosened further, changes will probably lead to substantial false-positive rates and unnecessary treatment. My advice to physicians is to use the DSM-5 cautiously, if at all. It is not an official manual."[244]

> It has long been argued that [the current] system of classifications makes unjustified categorical distinctions between disorders, and uses arbitrary cutoffs between normal and abnormal. A 2009 psychiatric review noted that attempts to demonstrate natural boundaries between related DSM syndromes, or between a common DSM syndrome and normality, have failed[245]

In a surprise announcement, "just two weeks before [the recent edition, the] *DSM-5* was due to appear, the National Institute of Mental Health, the world's largest funding agency for research into mental health, indicated that it is withdrawing support for the DSM manual. In a humiliating blow to the American Psychiatric Association, Thomas R. Insel, M.D., Director of the NIMH, made clear the agency would no longer fund research projects that rely exclusively on DSM criteria. Henceforth, the NIMH would be re-orienting its research away from DSM categories. 'The weakness' of the manual, [Dr. Insel] explained, 'is its lack of validity.

Unlike our definitions of ischemic heart disease [inadequate blood supply], lymphoma, or AIDS, the DSM diagnoses are based on a consensus about clusters of clinical symptoms, not any objective laboratory measure.' Insel pointed out: 'Symptom-based diagnosis, once common in other areas of medicine, has been largely replaced ... as we have understood that symptoms alone rarely indicate the best choice of treatment.[246] Too much of the DSM's earlier problems remain. The manual's precision and reliability has been overstated for decades.'"[247]

CLINICAL JUDGMENT

If we could agree that the essential question regarding a child's troublesome behavior is not what the child *has*, i.e., a disorder, but what the child *needs*, then clinical judgment is the *only* diagnostic procedure that allows a well-schooled professional to develop an answer and a suitable intervention.

While questionnaires, checklists and their numbers derived from the DSM represent the *least* valid and reliable assessment methods to determine if a child needs additional educational services, the most effective approach is by means of professional judgment as the psychologist can choose to:

- Evaluate the frequency and topography of a child's behavioral difficulties;
- Complete a functional assessment/analysis to determine the context (the who, what, when, where, and why) in which the troubling behaviors occur and do not occur, and, when trained in a broad spectrum; and
- Suggest possible remedial solutions that involve the child, the teacher, and the parent that go far beyond the use of medication.

In case you didn't notice, I intentionally avoided suggesting that a clinician should spend an exorbitant amount of time contemplating an ADHD diagnosis. An oft-repeated point, clinicians do not diagnosis ADHD. The fact remains that the clinicians can spend two hours or ten with kids, their families and their teachers gathering *critical* history in the privacy of their office, and they still won't meet ADHD face-to-face. At best, they'll log behaviors either observed directly (rarely), they'll learn time lines and behaviors' descriptions and frequencies within the context of home and/or school (all very important information), or they'll glean scattered information from parents' and teachers' problematic questionnaires, checklists, and rating scales. The clinician may even Ouija the DSM. And while there's potential value in the stem "Often doesn't seem to listen when spoken to directly," neither the stem nor the judgment "pretty much often" has anything to do with an organic diagnosis of ADHD.

Wherever clinicians place their professional faith, many will choose to fill out a form declaring ADHD as the official diagnosis. Unskilled readers of the form—insurance companies, the federal government's related administrators—will think the numbers real, just as they think ADHD is a real, biological disorder, rather than a convenient, one-dimensional acronym. If the only purpose for a medical model clinician's examination is to declare that a child *has* ADHD as a precursor to medication, then get it over fast, yes, "quick and dirty."

> One of the largest culprits of the entire controversy is our medical system's susceptibility to quick-and-dirty diagnoses,[248] exemplified by the fact that: doctors sometime prescribe Ritalin to children after just a fifteen minute evaluation.[249]

Why quick? The conclusion that the child has ADHD is *not* valid to begin with; what physician Michael Anderson judged was a trumped up exercise "to make something completely subjective look objective."[250]

The overburdened teacher, the obviously distraught parent, and/or the unsuccessful child are evidence enough that something needs to be done. Once the diagnostic exercise is completed, whether medication is prescribed or not, let the behaviorally trained clinician get to the important work at hand.

> "You definitely should be using behavior modification. You'll be giving your children much lower doses of medication over their lifetimes if you combine behavior modification with medication."[251]

- Establish the child's behavior at the data level, both the undesired *and* the desired alternatives (of which there will plenty).
- Determine when both the desired and undesired behaviors are most and least likely to occur.
- Determine what prompts the desired and undesired behaviors (looking closely at the curriculum assigned to the child).
- Determine how teachers and parents respond to the child's desired and undesired behaviors.

- Using the best clinical judgment, and in conjunction with a behavioral psychologist, determine what replicable interventions best fit the accumulated data, i.e., what the child needs, *never* medication solely but in conjunction with behavioral interventions, and suitable accommodations at school, which should be mandated without the need for a helium-filled ADHD diagnosis. There's nothing quick-and-dirty about any of that.

And while I'm at it, let's talk ADHD and profession roles. A physician's most important job is to rule out any unrecognized biological answer that might account for a child's undesired behavior, that and prescribing medication if it becomes necessary. Evaluating ADHD-like behaviors, however, is a task more suited to properly trained school-based or not office-bound behavioral psychologists, special education teachers, and speech and language pathologists. Physicians, with little chance to see a child at school or home, should leave the designations to those who observe the child in action and in context, where the greater part of the whole child acting within the greater part of the whole picture can be observed. In place of a contrived disorder, the active factors affecting the child are "diagnosed." From there, strategies flourish.

THE PARADOX

Except for a minority of cases involving distinct medical problems such as hyperthyroidism and explicit brain injuries, most youngsters diagnosed with ADHD may simply be normal, highly playful children who have difficulty adjusting to certain institutional expectations. ... [P]erhaps society should try to nurture this type of human variability or to adjust to it, rather than seeking to pathologize it and eliminate it with attention-focusing psychostimulants. It is certainly more rational to try to solve social problems with social solutions than with drugs, especially when the drugs are so similar to the ones we are trying to purge form our society.[252] (Jaak Panksepp, PhD, Emeritus Psychologist)

It is ironic that many who strongly resist ... prescription medication [for children] ... have no problem with using everyday stimulants to aid their own cognitive functioning.[253] According to Richard Rudgley,[254] "coffee, tea, cola, tobacco, and betel nut [are used] throughout the world to improve alertness and concentration in daily life." (Tom Brown, PhD, Psychologist)

[Add to Richard Rudgley's eye-openers "5-hour Energy" drink, recent annual sales about $1 billion; in 2011, 9 million bottles *a week*.][255,256]

When diagnosing the source of a problem, clinicians choose the simplest, most reliable, and most valid methodology possible, one that carries with it little controversy, one with an ease of application. If a medical issue is of central concern, the diagnosis best be biological, or at least biologically related.

As we've seen, three separate issues hamper an ADHD diagnosis. First, ADHD is not a biological entity. It's a representational construct. That precludes traditionally tried and verified diagnostic methodology such as those used to investigate cellular or chemical irregularities. Second, in place of instruments that measure biological components, diagnosticians are forced to rely on dubious data captured from questionnaires, checklists, and rating scales, and/or their own carefully considered judgment, which, according to some, isn't always reliable.

> Individual clinicians may not always recognize that errors in clinical judgment occur in their own practice. The core problem is that people are often poor at judging their own performance.[257] A related problem involves the tendency for people to form opinions on the basis of early information and, once these opinions are formed, their reluctance to change their opinions even when given important new information. Research in nonmedical settings suggests that experts are particularly prone to persevere with their initial ideas and to change their minds less frequently than would be ideal. Changing one's mind is unpleasant because it implies that the original thinking was incorrect. Changing one's mind in [clinical work] is even more troubling because of the need to explain the switch to patients, families, colleagues and others. A paradox also arises because clinical judgment is so cherished that it verges on being incorrigible.[258]

Third, and perhaps most importantly, an exploratory diagnostic investigation is enhanced significantly if the entity to be diagnosed is stable, somewhat predictable, easily defined, and clearly measurable. In the case of the medical model's ADHD, without genetic or neurological markers, we have none of the above. Instead, we're left exclusively with a child's behavior, as has been suggested.[259]

Taken as a whole, however, a child's behavior, unless operationalized and spoken of in data-level terms, suffers from a lack of definition that makes measurement difficult. Further, the child's behavior often has the nasty habit of changing itself with little notice, thereby offering little in the way of stability. Recall the well-behaved child in the clinician's office. Too bad the doctor didn't see the youngster the moment he got back into the family car on the way home. The clinician would have seen a different child. Medical physicians are fortunate their underlying contibutors, virus and bacteria, aren't so flighty.

But there was a moment in time when the medical model people influenced by the likes of Sir Alexander Crichton thought they had bagged lightning (or ADHD) in a bottle.

In the 1930s, psychiatrist Charles Bradley, working at a psychiatric asylum in Rhode Island, used the amphetamine Benzedrine in the 1930s to alleviate severe headaches and nausea induced when he drained young children's cerebrospinal fluid with a spinal tap.[260] The amphetamines did little to help the headaches or nausea but teachers at the Bradley home observed that it seemed to improve the ability of [children] to learn and behave in school.[261]

Much later,

Dozens of well-controlled studies showed that [stimulant] drugs immediately improved children's performance on repetitive tasks requiring concentration and diligence. Teachers and parents also reported improved behavior in almost every short-term study. Experts argued that because the brains of children with attention problems were different, the drugs had a mysterious paradoxical effect on them. This led many to conclude that the "brain deficit" hypothesis had been confirmed.[262]

And later still,

Some biological psychiatrists were puzzled by the fact that stimulants seemed paradoxically to calm hyperactive children, the belief in their effectiveness was such that ... stimulants were used as a diagnostic tool: if [stimulants] calmed down an over-active, impulsive child, then the child likely had hyperactivity.[263]

(FYI: Children don't *have* hyperactivity. The children may be described as "hyper," a subjective judgment that tells you very little about the child. "Energetic," "spirited," "frisky" also work. That's enough said.)

There it was. Proof. Documented. Historic. Authentic. The cause and solution were obvious. Under relatively controlled conditions, give a stimulant drug to a hyper, distractible child, the bane of all schoolteachers. Rather than hot-footing across the ceiling as one would expect a wired-child to do, if given a stimulating drug, many of the fidgety, inattentive bunch quieted. Some even focused and took a good shot at their school-work, though if they didn't know how to add to begin with, the stimulant medication didn't suddenly gift the children the needed wisdom to do so.

The transformation was spellbinding. The vocal majority had their bio-logical base. No longer the need to rely on a beleaguered teacher or par-ent's dogged pleas. Toss out the ratty questionnaires and checklists. Dump the much maligned DSM. A clinician's judgment? Not necessary. ADHD was a confirmed medical problem. Hyper child? Distracted child? No problem. No need to scrutinize the child in the context of his school day. No need to question a teacher's skills or a parent's management style when responding to the child's intolerable misbehavior. The child had a brain disorder. Administer Ritalin. "Cause" and "solution." Pretty much perfect. We got what we always wanted, a clear way to diagnose a malady, and, by darn, a pill.

Unfortunately, ever suspicious scientists don't sit idle when presented with a flagrant inconsistency, defined as anything that enters their ballpark wearing the wrap of an enigma. Hyper kids quieting down when given stimulants? Something's not kosher. These pestering people plead for per-plexing puzzles. And they're nasty, these scientists/egg-heads. Let the unsuspecting interloper with a wild idea venture out on a limb, somebody with a PhD's gonna fetch the chainsaw, always oiled and sharpened.

One of the old guys from Tom Brokaw's *Greatest Generation* remem-bered that "versions of these drugs had been given to World War II radar operators to help them stay awake and focus on boring, repetitive task."[264] That wasn't welcomed news. Radar operators couldn't have brain prob-lems. And one of the gals from the 1960s (another noted generation) remembered how these drugs improved memory and concentration, which was why they worked so well for college students cramming for exams. Uh-oh.

(FYI: Speaking of those once semi-exceptional 1950-60s college students, 90% (or thereabouts) of the then 20 year olds already knew that stimu-lants like coffee, tea, NoDoz, and especially chocolate could help a tired student keep his/her eyes open. Some of us, with a friendly physician available, discovered that what we called "horse-pills," which were huge 24-hour Dexedrine, time-released spansules, not only kept the con-sumer awake, the size-nine things opened a window to an inner brain that allowed whatever was crammed in to grab a chair and sit long enough to pass an exam. Sadly, after test-taking, while driving home or visiting a pub for a relaxing beer, if you tilted your head too far left or right, whatever you had stuffed into that brain of yours fell out your ears and into empty space. In other words, the acquisition was mostly short term unless practiced over time, what psychologists refer to as "space-trial learning," rather than "mass-trial-learning." Oh, the other 10% of those college students I referenced? The horse-pills put them to sleep. Not what you'd want during exam week.)

It was once thought you could diagnose the presence of ADHD by watching the effects of stimulant drugs. Thus, hyper children who calmed were thought to have ADHD. "We now know that nearly everyone who takes a low stimulant dosage stays alert and fidgets less."[265]

For years, it was assumed that stimulants had paradoxical calming effects in ADHD patients. It is now known that low doses of stimulants focus attention and improve executive function in both normal and ADHD subjects.[266]

Ugh! I won't ask the researcher how s/he decided who was and who wasn't ADHD. Yet again, stipulating "normal" versus "ADHD" subjects presumes we have a reliable, accurate means to know who's ADHD and who's not. In light of ADHD's inadequate diagnostic procedures, it's evident we have neither.

Biopsychiatry's researchers are aware that without proven diseases, ...the "disease" and "control" groups are ...indistinguishable. They know from the outset that their research is destined to prove nothing and to remain forever theoretical.[267]

"Stimulants ... tend to improve attention and reduce activity in all people, children and adults, irrespective of whether or not they are hyperactive." Author/psychologist Richard DeGrandpre posed the question: "Since most children 'benefit spectacularly' from taking Ritalin, does this mean that most of them also have ADD? Of course," not, he answered.[268]

(FYI: So you'll know, stimulant drugs don't take the place of good teachers and parents.)

"Medication helps a person be receptive to learning new skills and behaviors. But those skills and behaviors don't magically appear. They have to be taught," so advised psychologist Ruth Hughes.[269]

Hope Scott, a developmental pediatrician in Reston [Virginia], prescribes medication to most of her ADHD patients. But drugs are only one part of the plan. "Medications improve distractibility," Scott said. "But they do not touch development of time management or organizational skills. They help you focus on cleaning your room, but you still need to learn how to do it."[270]

A common misconception is that stimulants have a different effect on individuals with ADHD than they do on the general population. [Optional assignment. Try rewriting this entire paragraph without once mentioning ADHD, those supposedly with and those without. You'll make the same point in half the time and words.] This so-called paradoxical effect suggests that stimulants calm individuals with ADHD and energize people without ADHD. Because of this misconception, people reason that if a child's behavior improves after receiving medication, the diagnosis can be confirmed, but this is untrue. Children without ADHD respond to low doses of stimulant medication in the same way as children with ADHD. ... This suggests that stimulants do not have a paradoxical effect on children with ADHD and thus this reasoning cannot be used to verify a diagnosis.[271])

Beyond Diagnosis

ADHD "should not ever be used in our clinical thinking. ... Used as a primary diagnosis, 'ADHD' has no etiological significance. It is conceptually and diagnostically distracting; it leads to a paucity of thinking about a patient's early developmental history and trauma, and is therapeutically misleading."[272] (Claudia Gold MD, Pediatrician)

"There are no objective diagnostic criteria for ADHD."[273,274]

ADHD offers a unique platform upon which to try this open-minded, non-DSM-biased approach. Dropping the diagnosis of "ADHD" would have a number of advantages. It would encourage us to search more deeply for root causes; it would allow us to be more eclectic in our treatment; it would prevent patients, parents, doctors, teachers, and others from using it as a label or as an "excuse" for one's behavior; and it would require us to provide truly individualized care.[275] (Steve Balt, MD, Psychiatrist)

The hallmark symptoms of ADD/[ADHD]—distractibility, impulsivity, and high activity—are so commonly associated with children in general that the diagnosis is often not considered. ... How can we tell a spoiled child from an ADD child?[276] (Psychiatrists Edward Hallowell and John Ratey, from their book *Driven to Distraction*)

Frank Putnam, a director of one of NIMH's research units, applauded "the growing number of clinicians and researchers condemning the tyranny of our psychiatric and educational classification systems." Putnam found that it is exceedingly difficult to assign valid classifications to children, and yet "children are by far the most classified and labeled group in our society." He warned against "the institutional prescriptions of a system that seeks to pigeonhole them."[277]

Accepting ADHD as a real, genuine disorder supports the medical model's narrow interpretation. Inherent within the assumption is the belief that something's wrong with the child. It finger-points the youngster's genes and/or his or her neurology. Responsibility is inclusive *and* exclusive. It excuses everyone who has a say in the child's schooling, everyone and everything that does indeed contribute to the child's difficulties, however small, however unintended. The perspective portends poorly. What looms close should concern us all.

In an opinion piece entitled "Expand Pre-K, Not A.D.H.D.," written for the *New York Times*, researchers Stephen Hinshaw and Richard Scheffler acknowledged that "[t]he writing is on the chalkboard. Over the next few years, America can count on a major expansion of early childhood education. We embrace this trend, but as health policy researchers, we want to raise a major caveat: Unless we're careful, today's preschool bandwagon could lead straight to an epidemic of 4- and 5-year-olds wrongfully being told that they have [ADHD]." And they further point out that "[t]he problem is that millions of American children have been labeled … A.D.H.D. when they aren't." Their research revealed a "worrisome parallel between our nation's increasing push for academic achievement and increased school accountability—and skyrocketing A.D.H.D. diagnoses, particularly for the nation's poorest children."[278]

It's not as if this worry is just talk. Author and researcher Todd Elder working at Michigan State University reported that we're misdiagnosing our youngest children, the most behaviorally immature in their class. Elder said: "These children are significantly more likely than their older classmates to be prescribed behavior-modifying stimulants such as Ritalin. Such inappropriate treatment is particularly worrisome because of the unknown impacts of long-term stimulant use on children's health. It also wastes an estimated $320 million-$500 million a year on unnecessary medication—some $80 million-$90 million of it paid by Medicaid." Elder said the "smoking gun" of the study is that ADHD diagnoses depend on a child's age *relative to classmates* and the teacher's perceptions of whether the child has symptoms.

According to Elder's study, the youngest kindergartners were 60% more likely to be diagnosed with ADHD than the oldest children in the same grade. If a child is behaving poorly, if he's inattentive, if he can't sit still, it may simply be because he's 5 and the other kids are 6, so suggested Elder. ...Many ADHD diagnoses may be driven by teachers' perceptions of poor behavior among the youngest children in a kindergarten class-room. But these "symptoms" may merely reflect emotional or intellectual immaturity among the youngest students." (Emphases are mine.)[279]

> Structural and functional neuroimaging studies have not identified a unique etiology [for ADHD]. No genetic marker has been consistently identified, and heritability studies are confounded by familial environmental factors. The validity of the Conners Rating Scale-Revised has been seriously ques-tioned, and parent and teacher "ratings" of school children are frequently discrepant, suggesting that use of subjective information data via scale or interview does not form an objective basis for diagnosis of ADHD. Empirical diagnostic trials of stimulant medication that produces behavioral response have been shown not to distinguish between children with and without "ADHD." In summary, the working dogma that ADHD is a disease or neurobehavioral condition does not at this time hold up to scrutiny of evi-dence. Thorough evaluation of symptomatic children should be individual-ized, and include an assessment of educational, psychological, psychiatric, and family needs.[280]

> The "reliability" of a diagnosis refers to the degree to which it is depend-able; that is, the degree to which we can rely on the fact that the diagnosis will be the same regardless of who is doing the assessment or where the assessment is being done. For example, a broken arm is diagnosed through X-rays and there is a high likelihood that if you visited 100 orthopedic physi-cians with the same X-ray, all 100 would make the same diagnosis. "Broken arm" is a highly reliable diagnosis. In contrast, "ADHD" is an almost com-pletely *unreliable* diagnosis. "There are no objective diagnostic criteria for ADHD—no physical symptoms, no neurological signs, and no blood tests. … No physical test can be done to verify that a child has 'ADHD'."[281,282]

> The suggestion that 100 clinicians would likely come to no consensus on a child diagnosed by anyone as "ADHD" is borne out by the shocking dif-ferences in international prevalence rates. The prevalence of ADHD in the UK is generally estimated at 1% or less, whereas it is at least 10–12 times greater than that in Australia and the USA. This means that if you flew 12 "ADHD" children from Perth to London and had them assessed, the statistical likelihood is that only one would be a "confirmed" diagnosis. Factually,

then, the "disorder" is either grossly overdiagnosed in the USA, Australia, and Canada, or grossly underdiagnosed in the UK (and most of the rest of the world). In either case, it is not a diagnosis that can be depended upon; it lacks reliability.

Even *within* countries, wide variations in prevalence rates preclude the reliability of the diagnosis. For example, an analysis of the use of stimulant drugs for ADHD in the USA found that "Southern youngsters were about 71% more likely than kids in the Northeast or West to get the drugs, and Midwesterners were 51% more likely."[283]

MEDICATION: THE INEVITABLE DILEMMA

Because Ritalin to some extent sharpens focus and diminishes impulsivity in anyone, I must view it as [a] performance enhancer for everyone. ... Virtually all situations viewed as problems of inattention, impulse control, or hyperactivity will clinically improve with Ritalin use unless the picture includes a lot of anxiety, anger, or depression. ... The question I find myself asking most often is not who should get Ritalin, but who shouldn't.[284] (Lawrence H. Diller, MD, Developmental, Behavioral Pediatrician)

It's not uncommon for school personnel to seek medication to mitigate annoying/disorderly children under the guise of ADHD.

There's a tremendous push where if the kid's behavior is thought to be quote-unquote abnormal—if they're not sitting quietly at their desk—that's pathological, instead of just childhood.[285]

Overcrowded classrooms, little immediate support from school administration, changes in curriculum standards, all represent a much broader system problem, and teachers are frequently the ones who unfairly bear the blame. Sometimes medication is the only alternative, they'll tell you. That granted, the diagnosis of ADHD, with its resulting medication, comes with serious problems related to what psychologists call "best practice."

Peter Breggin, psychiatrist, says that "By making an A.D.H.D. diagnosis, we ignore and stop looking for what is really going on with the child."[286]

Some physicians counter saying that short-term relief provided by medication can obscure a child's underlying psychological and environmental problems and prevent them from being closely examined. "We're pouring some water on the fire, and my concern is we're never going back to see why the fire got started."[287] (David Rubin, Pediatrician)

Psychiatrist Sidney Walker III, MD says: "The medical community has elevated Attention Deficit Disorder (ADD) and Attention Deficit Hyperactivity Disorder (ADHD) to the status of diagnoses, and most people believe these are real diseases. They aren't, and doctors who label children ADD or ADHD don't have a clue what's really ailing them."[288]

Recall CHADD's statement regarding ADHD being a "hidden disability": "ADD is not hard to spot. Just look with your eyes and listen with your ears when you walk through places where children are—particularly those places where children are expected to behave in a quiet, orderly, and productive fashion. In such places, children ... will identify themselves quite readily." As pointed out, the annoyed teachers were *not* observing ADHD. They were observing children adapting to the context within which they found themselves. That the children did annoy the teachers should have been a sign the educators used to alter their curriculum and management approaches. They chose not to, believing the children were impaired. Today, it's easy to suggest a child *has* a disorder. Teachers notify parents, questionnaires are filled out, the information is provided to a physician, and both the diagnosis and resulting medication are forthcoming, often promptly.

There's a downside to this expedient, often first-choice approach. Consider the medical model's tenets (Box 4.9).

Box 4.9   Medical model

Short of swallowing pills, the **Medical** model does not require that a youngster be a part of the solution.

The **Medical** model requires little in the way of a child, or his/her teacher's, active involvement.

The **Medical** model relies on drugs to solve problems *passively*.

"Learned helplessness" clearly becomes a possibility. Recall the young boy who told the interviewer: "Without my drugs, I'd have an attitude. I'd be disrespectful to my parents."[289] The youngster was unlikely to learn anything positive from the "therapeutic" intervention since his only participation was swallowing pills, and his parents' only responsibility was to watch the clock.

Psychoactive drugs eroded the ability of groups and individuals to "make provisions and develop strategies of human relatedness, which serve to regulate … anxiety, grief, rage, and more extreme forms of behavior. In other words, such drugs acted as a crutch, preventing children from developing their own strategies to cope with their academic and behavior shortcomings."[290]

For the easily convinced, ADHD tells the significant adults in the child's life that the problem is the child's. By default, it tells the child that he or she is disabled. It tells the youngster that drugs will do for him what he can't do himself. With that attitude, the problem will become the child's—and his parents' if by chance the child should falter. Intervention is limited to varied or increased dosages of medication, the results mixed as to the long-term effects.[291,292,293,294,295] Not surprisingly, the child may carry those dependent lessons into his or her future. The message the child hears, "Honey, there's something wrong with your brain and this little pill's going to fix everything."[296] Today, the mom being interviewed was *that* child. The experience those many years earlier was not one she valued.

> The persistent search for a biological cause of ADD over the past decade has led me reluctantly to conclude that psychiatric academia appears more interested in the environment of the synapse than in the environment of the child.[297]

Medical practitioners who know brains and chemistry search out what they see as related pathologies, e.g., brain anomalies and chemical/genetic deviations. Consequently, they are inclined to use different chemistry to alter children's brains—a narrow view if that's all they do. They treat ADHD as a medical challenge, a problem involving brain chemistry. They offer as evidence that certain drugs help kids with ADHD-like symptoms improve their performance in school. We know, of course, that the drugs can assist most kids, assuming they have a good teacher and the right curriculum. Even then, numerous kids over the years have come to me and begged me to get them off their medication, complaining that it interfered with their lives. The best I could do was to suggest they speak to their parents.

I'm quick to voice strong opposition to this medical approach involving school-related issues. It's equivalent to considering the personality of a sea star (starfish) by looking at only one of its many arms. Once again, ADHD-like behavior is best viewed initially *not* as a medical problem, but as an educational challenge suited to special educators and behavioral trained psychologists and speech and language pathologists whose relevant evaluation and (nonmedical) intervention skills are far superior to those held by traditionally trained, office-bound physicians without any developmental and/or behavioral background. You have the option to disagree. Let me try to convince you otherwise.

NIMH, a highly respected government organization, is the largest research organization in the world specializing in mental illness. Though their credentials are without equal, they're not immune to mistakes, particularly with respect to ADHD.

The following statement from NIMH highlights their narrow brain-chemical approach to ADHD. It's like they wrote their position three decades ago and saw no reason to dust it off.

Their etiological position states that:

"ADHD probably results from a combination of factors."[298]

The qualifier "probably" makes the statement embarrassingly safe and noncommittal. I'd expect more from the government's major mental health agency. NIMH tells us:

Scientists are not sure what causes ADHD, although many studies suggest that genes play a large role. Like many other illnesses, ADHD probably results from a combination of factors. In addition to genetics, researchers are looking at possible environmental factors, and are studying how brain injuries, nutrition, and the social environment might contribute to ADHD.[299]

I wasn't surprised by NIMH's inclusion of "brain injuries" and "nutrition," both biologics certainly worthy of consideration as factors affecting a child's *behavior* while attending school. But I was pleasantly surprised, actually ecstatic, that NIMH acknowledged "environmental factors" and even mentioned the "social environment."

Unfortunately, the words "environment" and "social environment" are constructs requiring that I speculate what NIMH meant by their use. Because of my background, I assumed "environment" comprised the total life space within which a child lived and developed. I assumed it included parents, siblings, dogs, cats, aunts, uncles, cousins, teachers and curriculum and classrooms, home support, family style, motivation, attitudes and interest, TV, movies, books, electronic everything, music, soccer, baseball, among five dozen other interrelated, and interdependent, dynamics that occur most every day in a child's ever-changing, challenging life. I made that assumption. I thought it was one of those, you know, "no brainers." I mean, we're talking about a child's environment. Right?

Boy, was I wrong. NIMH stayed true to its restrictive medical model calling, specifically its penchant for brains and chemistry and nothing else. You'd think one of their experts would have had a broader education. I read with utter dismay NIMH's insular "Environmental Factors":

> Studies suggest a potential link between cigarette smoking and alcohol use during pregnancy and ADHD in children. In addition, preschoolers who are exposed to high levels of lead, which can sometimes be found in plumbing fixtures or paint in old buildings, may have a higher risk of developing ADHD.[300]

There's your medical model's anemic environmental answer to the question "Why is my child struggling in school?" No mention of a child's daily living experiences, current and/or historical. As I read NIMH's unique interpretation on what the environment represents, I wondered what options their view offered a worried mom or dad with a five-year-old who met ADHD criteria? Brains and chemistry—that's all NIMH offered. That's sad.

NIMH's claims are standard oratory. They're equivalent to the pre-Copernicus, pre-Galileo fifteenth-century sun that the church insisted revolved around the earth. It's ignorance, and no manner of authoritative edict will alter that inadequacy. As weak as NIMH's etiological statement is, "ADHD probably results from a combination of factors...," it's still incorrect. The construct ADHD is not a measurable effect or a physical, quantifiable outcome. It does not result from a combination of factors. It's a crafted, voted upon name, an umbrella, a bridge, a convenient representational construct, one that stands together with other representational constructs such as pneumonia, learning disabilities, cerebral palsy, and dyslexia. There's nothing wrong with any of the terms so long as they stay where they belong, as paltry adjectives used to describe, and not as part of a correlational or causative statement where we wrongly force them to be what they aren't: physical entities with independent, biologic properties.

At the least, NIMH's position statement *should* read:

> "A child's problematic behaviors, often interpreted as signs of a mental health disorder, result from a combination of factors. Involved elements include the child's brain, the child's chemistry, the child's genetics, and to a substantial extent the child's everyday, social and familial environment that

continuously integrates countless variables and their multiple interactions. Along with given temperament, these environmentally produced interactions have contributed to the youngster's behavioral, emotional, and intellectual history from the time of the child's birth. The supposition that genes or neurology alone or in large measure account for the complex behaviors associated with the construct ADHD is neither sound nor supported. It's time to recognize the child's exhibited behaviors as effects of numerous biologic and ongoing environmental influences, and that medication, to the exclusion of other interventions that focus on family systems, represents not only a weak approach to remediation, but a medical disservice to a child and the child's family."

The medical model and its narrow perspective and treatment dominate professional thinking regarding ADHD. It's helpful to hear alternative voices. You might find this worthwhile. Robert Whitaker is a prominent medical writer whose concentration is on psychiatric care and psychotropic drugs. In this presentation, he provides important information about how ADHD—now an "epidemic"—is diagnosed and why users of medications for ADHD should be cautious. Recent news stories about the hazards of long-term ADHD medications and the more general use of these drugs to enhance concentration underscore the importance of Whitaker's discussion.[301] See:

http://www.scienceforthepublic.org/medical-research/medicating-adhd-diagnosis-and-the-long-term-effects-of-the-medications/

By good fortune, I happened upon this message from many years past, approaching a half-century, and thought it too topical not to add to our discussion. The Representative (and father) was well ahead of his time.

Representative Cornelius Gallaher September 29, 1970, Hearing of the House of Representatives: hearing into Federal responsibility in promoting the use of amphetamines to modify the behavior of grammar schoolchildren. Representative Gallagher said:

As a father of four, I am well aware of the occasional frustrations which come from the fact that children do not simply sit quietly and perform assigned tasks. Based on my personal experience, I believe that children learn with all their senses, not just with the eyes and ears. For childhood is an exploratory time and the great energy of children propels them into situations which may look frivolous or counterproductive to more restrained adults, but which are the sum and substance of the child's learning experience. I do not think I am overstating the case when I say that the learning environment for the young child is the total environment and every experience is a learning experience. Obviously, this unstructured passion for all the events in a child's world is regarded as unruly and disruptive, particularly in overcrowded classrooms. I fear that there is a very great temptation to diagnose the bored but bright child as hyperactive, prescribe drugs, and thus deny him full learning during his most creative years.[302]

Speaking poignantly, Lawrence H. Diller, from his book, *Running On Ritalin* shared his own musings. "My awareness of the pressures on parents and children is always with me as I evaluate for ADD. ... There's little I can do to change the big picture: I can't reduce class sizes, nor increase funding for public education. ... I can, however, address as many remedial factors as possible. ... And, in the end, I can help this child ... cope a bit better by offering him Ritalin."

"Still, this doesn't seem enough," Diller continued. "As far back as 1980, ... [psychologists and authors] Carol Whalen and Barbara Hencker discussed the 'social trap' doctors face when they prescribe Ritalin for a child.[303] While the physician may be 'doing good,' on an individual basis, they note, by enhancing the child's performance with medication, he or she may unwittingly be contributing to a 'social bad.' It's a well-known conundrum of child psychiatry that even an effective psychopharmacological intervention may permit a poor environment to continue or worsen. When American doctors distribute fifteen tons of Ritalin to children in just one year, are they accepting and abetting the fact of overcrowded classrooms, overwhelmed parents and teachers, and unreasonable standards?"[304]

Active kids who have been mislabeled with ADHD suffer unnecessary stigma, reduced expectations, and harmful drug side effects. We need to do a better job of protecting our children from such widespread careless diagnosis and reckless treatment. ... Our country is spending far too much on unnecessary and often ... harmful medical care and far too little on education. It is completely irrational to shortchange our schools and then spend a bundle on misguided medical treatment for normally active kids who don't do well in a stressed school environment. [We'd do] better if most of [our] misspent and wasted money were instead budgeted toward better schools. We should be able to manage the more active kids with educational tools rather than subjecting them to fake medical diagnoses.[305] (Allen Frances, MD, Psychiatrist)

Schools

The authors of the study hypothesized that increased demands in school are leading to a rise in the diagnosis of ADHD. In order to answer this question, they first looked at studies that documented the time children spent on academic activities in the U.S. since 1970. Not surprisingly, they found that the time spent on academic activities has increased dramatically for children. This is particularly true for pre-school aged children who are being exposed to reading and writing activities much earlier than in the past. The researchers did end up finding that as academic demands and homework increased, so did rates of [diagnosed] ADHD.[306]

Schools change children. Their first order of business is to take diverse youngsters and slowly but inexorably sculpt them until they're like one another. Parris Island in South Carolina does the same with new Marine recruits, though the DIs [Drill Instructors] accomplish the transformation in 24 hours or less.

Because of the way we assemble our classrooms with one teacher and roughly 30 diverse kids, where curriculum is preplanned and served in one package, the effort at standardizing pupils is necessary, though it is often ineffective. One teacher and 25–35 kids together in a tight cubicle, no matter how colorful the walls and ceiling, puts a damper on individualized teaching. The ratio doesn't eliminate tailored instruction, but it does strangle away most of its oxygen. The task is particularly challenging with K-5 kids:

- All with different temperament juices flowing
- All with different brains maturing
- All with environmental history forming

A crowded classroom? Jonathan Swift's "old lady in a shoe" has her work cut out.

We live in a world that is highly competitive, an intense world that greets our children from the first days of kindergarten. Look at their curriculum; look at what we ask them to do; look at the pressures their parents find themselves facing. There's a must-succeed mentality that places great strain on patience, understanding, differences, and deviations, and being as good as someone else. It's prime for the medical model: it's a fabricated petri dish where discrepancies grow with amazing speed, so much so that medical doctors are ready to medicate three-year-olds for what amounts to a contrived condition.[307]

Variations among schoolchildren always amaze. Beyond hair color and dress, contrasting aspects of the children strike you instantly:

- Their language
- Their animation
- Their intensity
- Their attending
- Their entering skills
- Their acquired manners and consideration
- Their outward expressions of emotions
- The way they take to a group with confidence
- The way they slip quietly into a corner and watch the new world with flat, perhaps wary, expressions

Dynamic portraits of remarkable individual differences on display, easily lost when the medical model flexes.

But we can only know what a child shows us, the smallest portion of the youngster, the equivalent to an outcropping's nose. To fully appreciate a child's total uniqueness, we must add to the mix the youngster's acquired tendencies, his genetic leanings, his brain capabilities, and his persuasive history all of which constantly interact. More still. Each child possesses inherent physical, artistic, and cognitive strengths, weaknesses, and limits, most known only when they exhibit themselves—or fail to do so. Further, each child enters school with needs, drives, attitudes, purpose, motivations, worries and fears, hopes and dreams, though no two children come with the same of each, either in fact or in established priority. Each child who enters school brings along challenges, some obvious, some subtle, some easily resolved, some with great urgency. Each child represents the quintessential self, different now, destined different forever.

It's when we toy with that self, wanting or expecting it to be another self, that problems surface and talk of developmental inappropriateness rises. Of all places, yet, in school, with our youngsters still finding their footing, we speak so casually, so quickly of disorders the young child has. ADHD, the child must have. How else can we explain that s/he is different from others, so *not* what *is* normal. Small of us, I think.

The concept of normality has no place, certainly not in schools. If natural normality has no place, then neither does natural abnormality. The only child-abnormality that exists is that which we fabricate for some purpose— as an easy answer, to codify, to end a conversation, to make ourselves money. Extending a child a helping hand does not require the concept of abnormality. A child even in minor discomfort is sufficient justification for the therapist to apply his or her skills. A child in major pain should have been attended to much earlier. But for insurance company's purposes, a psychiatric stamp that declares "defective" is unnecessary. ADHD, no matter what we say it is or isn't, does not—cannot—stand on its own. ADHD has no skeleton, no skin, no heart. It requires comparison before a contrived diagnosis can be made. To be diagnosed, and thus be given an invisible footprint, it needs more than one child. That should say enough for us to either discard it, or get it over with quickly.

What should we be diagnosing? How a child compares to other children? Why? We don't choose interventions based on what other children do, but what the child in question does in the context in which the behaviors occur.

In school, the initial diagnostic questions remain:

- Does the child's behavior interfere with his or her ability to learn?
- Does the child interfere with other student's ability to learn?
- Does the child interfere with a teacher's ability to teach?

If a child meets any of these criteria, the initial diagnostic procedure confirms the child needs *assistance*. Behaviorally trained psychologists and special education teachers know what steps to take. Does being told that a child was diagnosed ADHD tell anyone what to do? Resoundingly, "No." In fact, the construct serves as a hindrance. It's like a faulty weathervane; it points the remedial team (including the child's parents) in the wrong direction.

Consigning the ADHD decision to professionals who espouse the pathologically driven, medical model provides few options for treatment strategies. Odds are that the child exhibiting persistent behavior and attention problems in school will be diagnosed ADHD and will be placed on medication. The context within which the child functions will be ignored, Sir Alexander Crichton's uninformed thesis that the problem is always the child winning out. Medical model people are rarely trained to consider much else.

Most likely, medication will change the child's chemistry and perhaps his or her behavior, though not by anything active the child has done, not anything active that would teach the child how to ultimately direct himself. But it will not directly change anything else that *contributes* to the child's difficulties, not what's contributed (inadvertently) by the parents, not what's contributed (inadvertently) by the child's school or its teachers. That which maintains the undesired behavior will remain, ready to cause trouble if the unknowing child should falter.

Seriously missing from the ADHD equation is any discussion centered on what and who, besides the child, needs modifying. Left to the medical model, the answer is always the child's executive brain. Left to that, false positives—children said to be disordered who are not—are guaranteed.

Let's end our discussion where we began, the continual debate that remains open, inviting you to find your place within (Box 4.10).

Box 4.10   ADHD

The American Academy of Pediatrics, American Medical Association, American Psychiatric Association, and National Institutes of Health recognize ADHD as a valid condition.[a]	"ADHD seems to have become more or less the catchall designation for children who do not 'behave well'."[b]

[a]http://www.webmd.com/add-adhd/childhood-adhd/features/adhd-critics#1
[b]http://articles.mercola.com/sites/articles/archive/2013/07/20/drugging-children.aspx

---

Perhaps John Merrow's 1995 PBS report "ADD—A Dubious Diagnosis" will help you select which side of this debate seems more to your liking. It is your class assignment. I assure you it will not leave you neutral.

https://www.youtube.com/watch?v=eMNhdvg8kgA

NOTES

1. Levine, P. (February 26, 2014). Francis Bacon on confirmation bias. *peterlevine.ws*. Retrieved from http://peterlevine.ws/?p=13386.
2. http://www.pbs.org/wgbh/pages/frontline/shows/medicating/interviews/barkley.html
3. Breggin, P. (2001) *Talking back to Ritalin: What doctors aren't telling you about stimulants for children.* (pp. 147, 179). Cambridge, MA: Da Capo Press.
4. https://www.healthcentral.com/article/addadhd-is-fiction-not-a-real-disease#sthash.411hpBry.dpuf
5. http://www.nytimes.com/roomfordebate/2011/10/12/are-americans-more-prone-to-adhd/adhd-is-a-misdiagnosis

6. http://www.chadd.org/understanding-adhd/about-adhd/the-science-of-adhd.aspx

7. http://www.snopes.com/politics/quotes/adhd.asp/

8. http://www.pbs.org/wgbh/pages/frontline/shows/medicating/interviews/koplewicz.html

9. John S. Werry, M.D., Emeritus Professor of Psychiatry, Head, Department of Psychiatry, School of Medicine, University of Auckland (New Zealand). See Diller, L.H. (1998) *Running on Ritalin: A physician reflects on children, society, and performance in a pill*. New York: Bantam. p. 101.

10. Barkley, Russel (2010). *ADHD in adults: What the science says*. New York: The Guilford Press. p. 435.

11. Fine, L. (2001, May 9). Paying attention: Scientists scrutinize the brain for biological clues to the mysteries of ADHD. *Education Week*, 26–29; MSNBC, 2000--MSNBC. (2000, December 16). *Brain scan may help diagnose ADHD*. http://www.msnbc.com/news/347444.asp

12. NIH Consensus Report, 1998–National Institutes of Health Consensus Statement. (1998, November). *Diagnosis and treatment of attention deficit hyperactivity disorder.*

13. Hinshaw, S.P., & Scheffler, R.M. (2014). *The ADHD Explosion: Myths, Medication, Money, and Today's Push for Performance*. (p. 99) New York: Oxford University Press.

14. Hinshaw, S.P., & Scheffler, R.M. (p. 101).

15. Rutgers professor David Mechanic writing in the foreword to Hinshaw, S.P., & Scheffler, R.M. (2014).

16. http://www.collective-evolution.com/2016/09/01/adhd-is-a-fake-disorder-says-neurologist-turned-author/

17. http://abcnews.go.com/Health/Healthday/brain-studies-show-adhd-real-disease/story?id=4508193

18. Gil Anaf, Oral Testimony to the South Australia Parliamentary Committee Inquiry into Attention Deficit Hyperactivity Disorder, *Hansard*, August 24, 2001, p. 61.

19. https://www.psychologytoday.com/blog/child-in-mind/201608/big-pharma-and-the-question-is-adhd-real

20. Conners C.K. The computerized continuous performance test. Psychopharmacol Bull. 1985; 21:891–892. [PubMed].

21. Hinshaw, S.P., & Scheffler, R.M. p. xxv.

22. McGuiness, D. (1989). Attention deficit disorder: The emperor's clothes, animal "pharm," and other fiction. In S. Fischer & R.P. Greenberg (Eds.), *The limits of biological treatments for psychological distress: Comparisons with psychotherapy and placebo* (p. 155). Hillsdale, NJ: Erlbaum.

23. See "Comments." https://www.nytimes.com/roomfordebate/2011/10/12/are-americans-more-prone-to-adhd/adhd-is-a-misdiagnosis

24. Bart, S. (February 8, 2012). Why we should eliminate the diagnosis of ADHD. *Conditions.* See http://www.kevinmd.com/blog/2012/02/eliminate-diagnosis-adhd.html

25. Barkley, R., Cook, E., Dulcan, M., Campbell, S., Prior, M., Gillberg, M., Solanto-Gardner, M., Halperin, J., Bauermeister, J., Pliszka, S., Stein, M., Werry, J., Brown, R. (2002). Consensus Statement on ADHD. *European Journal of Child and Adolescent Psychiatry, 11*(2), 96–98.

26. Hinshaw, S. P., & Scheffler, R.M. (2014) p.29.

27. Patino, E. (2016). Chiropractic therapy: What it is and how it works. *understood.org.* Retrieved from https://www.understood.org/en/learning-attention-issues/treatments-approaches/alternative-therapies/chiropractic-therapy-what-it-is-and-how-it-works.

28. Patino, E. (2016).

29. DeGrandpre, R. (1999). *Ritalin Nation.* New York: W.W. Norton & Company; Smith, M. (2012). *Hyperactive: The controversial history of ADHD.* Reaktion Books; http://www.amazon.com/Attention-Deficit-Disorder-Natural-Alternatives-Therapy/dp/1553120329; see: Buttross, S.L. (2007). *Understanding attention deficit hyperactivity disorder.* Jackson MS: University Press of Mississippi.

30. Smith, J. (2017). ADD/ADHD: Kids Being Over-Diagnosed and Over-Medicated? *empowher.org.* Retrieved from http://www.empowher.com/attention-deficit-hyperactivity-disorder-adhd/content/addadhd-kids-being-over-diagnosed-and-over-med.

31. Reinberg, S. (Tuesday, September 4, 2007). 9% of U.S. kids have ADHD. *Health day reporter.* Retrieved from http://www.washingtonpost.com/wpdyn/content/article/2007/09/03/AR2007090300729.html.

32. Smith, J. (2017).

33. Reinberg, S. (Tuesday, September 4, 2007).

34. Gualtiere, C.T., & Johnson, L.G. (2005 Nov). *ADHD: Is objective diagnosis possible?* Psychiatry, 2(11), pp. 44–53.

35. Henion, A., & Elder, T. (August 17, 2010). Nearly 1 million children potentially misdiagnosed with ADHD. *msutoday,msu.edu.* http://msutoday.msu.edu/news/2010/nearly-1-million-children-potentially-misdiagnosed-with-adhd/.

36. Schwarz, A. & Cohen, S. (2013, March 31). A.D.H.D. Seen in 11% of U.S. children as diagnoses rise. Retrieved from http://www.nytimes.com/2013/04/01/health/more-diagnoses-of-hyperactivity-causing-concern.html?pagewanted%253Dall&_r=0.

37. Hinshaw, S.P., & Scheffler, R.M. (2014), p. 137.

38. Elizabeth, R. (August 16, 2013). Signs of ADHD in a 2-year-old. *livestrong.com.* Retrieved from http://www.livestrong.com/article/512541-signs-of-adhd-in-a-2-year-old/.

39. Bailey, E. (2017). ADHD in children: Birth through 12 months. *health-central.com*. Retrieved from http://www.healthcentral.com/adhd/raising-child-with-adhd-278672-5_2.html; http://www.healthcentral.com/adhd/raising-child-with-adhd-278672-5.html.
40. Center for disease control. (March 31, 2017). Attention Deficit Hyperactivity Disorder (ADHD). *cdcgov*. Retrieved from http://www.cdc.gov/nchs/fastats/adhd.htm.
41. Hatfield, R. (January 16, 2014). Top ADHD medications. *livestrong.com*. Retrieved from http://www.livestrong.com/article/68947-top-ten-adhd-medications/.
42. Schwarz, A. (2014, May 16). Thousands of Toddlers Are Medicated for A.D.H.D., Report Finds, Raising Worries. *nytimes.com*. Retrieved from https://www.nytimes.com/2014/05/17/us/among-experts-scrutiny-of-attention-disorder-diagnoses-in-2-and-3-year-olds.html?smid=pl-share&_r=1.
43. Handelman, K. (November 30, 2012). Are ADHD meds safe. *Huffingtonpost.ca*. Retrieved from http://www.huffingtonpost.ca/dr-kenny-handelman/adhd_b_1925852.html.
44. Reuters. (May 5, 2014) Long-term safety of ADHD medicine still a question, study says. *foxnews.com*. Retrieved from http://www.foxnews.com/health/2014/05/05/long-term-safety-adhd-medicine-still-question-study-says/.
45. Harrison, P. (July 17, 2014). ADHD drugs not tested for safety, efficacy over time. *medscape.com*. Retrieved from http://www.medscape.com/viewarticle/828445.
46. Harrison, P. (July 17, 2014).
47. Schwarz, A. & Cohen, S. (2013, March 31).
48. Hallowell, E.M. (May–June 1997). "What I've learned from ADD." *Psychology Today*, 41–44.
49. Gordon, M., Barkley, R.A., & Murphy, K. (August 1997) "ADHD on Trial," *ADHD Report*, vol. t, pp. 1–4.
50. Paterno, D. (2010). *Why your child needs a parent in charge and how to become one*. Bloomington, IN: WestBow Press.
51. Gold, C. (2013). We need a movement to deconstruct the ADHD diagnosis. kevinmd.com. Retrieved from http://www.kevinmd.com/blog/2013/12/movement-deconstruct-adhd-diagnosis.html.
52. D.J. Morrow. (September 2, 1997). Attention Disorder Is Found in Growing Number of Adults, *New York Times*, D4. Retrieved from http://www.nytimes.com/1997/09/02/business/attention-disorder-is-found-in-growing-number-of-adults.html.
53. Author Elizabeth. (Jan 18, 2017). Renowned Harvard psychologist says ADHD is largely a fraud. *curiousmindmagazine.com* Retrieved from http://curiousmindmagazine.com/harvard-psychologist-says-adhd-largely-fraud/

54. http://www.cdc.gov/nchs/fastats/adhd.htm
55. Schwarz, A. (Oct 9, 2012). Attention disorder or not, pills to help in school. *nytimes.com.* Retrieved from http://www.nytimes.com/2012/10/09/health/attention-disorder-or-not-children-prescribed-pills-to-help-in-school.html?_r=0.
56. Baughman, F. (May 4, 2000). Medicating kids. Interview Frontline PBS. *pbs.org.* Retrieved from http://www.pbs.org/wgbh/pages/frontline/shows/medicating/interviews/baughman.html
57. Berezin, R. (March 17, 2015). No, there is no such thing as ADHD. *madinamerica.com.* Retrieved from http://www.madinamerica.com/2015/03/no-no-thing-adhd/
58. Jensen, P. (September 12, 2000). Medicating kids. Interview Frontline PBS. *pbs.org.* Retrieved from http://www.pbs.org/wgbh/pages/frontline/shows/medicating/interviews/jensen.html.
59. Kurtz, S. (May 09, 2012). What is ADHD, and why do people say it doesn't exist? *Huffingtonpost.com.* Retrieved from http://www.huffingtonpost.com/2012/05/09/what-is-adhd_n_1500294.html
60. Adesman, A.R. (2001) The diagnosis and management of attention-deficit/hyperactivity disorder in pediatric patients. *ncbi.nlm.nih.gov.* Retrieved from http://www.ncbi.nlm.nih.gov/pmc/articles/PMC181164/
61. Schwarz, A. (May 6, 2014).
62. Goodman, B. (2014). Minority kids less likely to get ADHD diagnosis? *webmd.com.* Retrieved from http://www.webmd.com/add-adhd/childhood-adhd/news/20130624/minority-kids-less-likely-to-be-diagnosed-treated-for-adhd-study
63. Gladwell, M. (February 2, 1999) Running from Ritalin. *gladwell.com.* Retrieved from http://gladwell.com/running-from-ritalin/
64. Diller, L.H. (1998) *Running on Ritalin: A physician reflects on children, society, and performance in a pill.* (p. 49) New York: Bantam.
65. Milich R., Pelham W.E., Hinshaw S.P. Issues in the diagnosis of attention deficit disorder: A cautionary note on the Gordon Diagnostic System. *Psychopharmacol Bull.* 1986; 22:1101–1104. [PubMed].
66. Power T.J., Contextual factors in vigilance testing of children with ADHD. *J Abnorm Child Psychol.* 1992; 20:579–593. [PubMed].
67. Block, M. (n.d.) *No more ADHD.* (p. 10) Hurst, TX: Block System Publishers.
68. Diller, L.H. (1998), (p. 60).
69. Baughman, F.A. (2002) Untitled blog. *psychrights.org.* Retrieved from http://psychrights.org/research/Digest/ADHD/ADHDAsFraud.htm
70. Hallahan, D.P.; Kauffman, J.M. (2005) *Exceptional learners: Introduction to special education.* Boston: Allyn & Bacon.

71. Moffitt, T.E., & Melchior, M. (2007, Jun). Why does the worldwide prevalence of childhood attention deficit hyperactivity disorder matter? *Am J Psychiatry, 164*(6):856–8.
72. Paterno, D. (2010).
73. Amaral, O.B. (2007, Oct). Psychiatric disorders as social constructs: ADHD as a case in point. *Am J Psychiatry, 164*(10):1612; author reply 1612–3.
74. Taylor, E. (1989). *On the epidemiology of hyperactivity. In attention deficit disorder: clinical and basic research.* Hillsdale: N.J., Lawrence Erlbaum Associates. pp. 31–52, 31.
75. Diller, L.H. (1998). (p. 193).
76. Hallowell, E.M. (May–June 1997).
77. Duperret, N. (2000) Medicating kids: four families, four children. Frontline PBS. *pbs.org.* http://www.pbs.org/wgbh/pages/frontline/shows/medicating/four/
78. Schwarz, A. (Oct 9, 2012).
79. Gunsberg, J. (October 24, 2012) Giving Adderall to poor children who don't have ADHD. Retrieved from http://www.losangelesjuveniledefense.com/giving-adderall-to-poor-children-who-dont-have-adhd/
80. Bernstein, L. (April 1, 2015). Nearly half of all preschoolers with ADHD are on medication. *washingtonpost.com.* Retrieved from https://www.washingtonpost.com/news/to-your-health/wp/2015/04/01/nearly-half-of-all-pre-schoolers-with-adhd-are-on-medication/?utm_term=.3b02bb2ac5b9
81. Iannelli, V. (March 14, 2011) The history and medication timeline of ADHD. *verywell.com.* Retrieved from http://pediatrics.about.com/od/adhd/a/history_adhd.htm
82. Hinshaw, S.P., & Scheffler, R.M. (2014) p. 6.
83. Simon, B. (February 24, 2015) ADHD medication prescriptions are off the charts—Why? and should we be worried. *Inquisitr.com* Retrieved from http://www.inquisitr.com/1871461/adhd-medication-prescriptions-are-off-the-charts-why-and-should-we-be-worried/
84. Number of Children & Adolescents Taking Psychiatric Drugs in the U.S. (2017). *cchrint.org.* Retrieved from https://www.cchrint.org/psychiatric-drugs/children-on-psychiatric-drugs/
85. Hersch, C. The Clinician and the Joint Commission Report: A Dialogue. *Journal of the American Academy of Child Psychiatry, 10* (1971)', p. 411.
86. The history of ADHD: A timeline. (n.d.) healthline.com. Retrieved from http://www.healthline.com/health/adhd/history#overview1
87. Burd L., Kerbeshian J. Historical roots of ADHD. J Am Acad Child Adolesc Psychiatry. 1988; 27:262. doi:10.1097/00004583-198803000-00021. [PubMed].

88. Klaus, W.L., Reichi, S., Lange, K.M., Tucha, L., & Tucha, O. (December 2010). The history of attention deficit hyperactivity disorder. *ncbi.nlm. nih.gov.* Retrieved from https://www.ncbi.nlm.nih.gov/pmc/articles/ PMC3000907/

89. Crichton, A. (1798). *An Inquiry Into the Nature and Origin of Mental Derangement: Comprehending a Concise System of the Physiology and Pathology of the Human Mind. And a History of the Passions and Their Effects,* p. 272; 278.

90. History of attention deficit hyperactivity disorder. (n.d.) *en.wikipedia.org.* Retrieved https://en.wikipedia.org/wiki/History_of_attention_deficit_ hyperactivity_disorder

91. Crichton, A. (1798).

92. Crichton, A. (1798).

93. History of attention deficit hyperactivity disorder. (n.d.) Retrieved December 10, 2015 from Wikipedia https://en.wikipedia.org/wiki/ History_of_attention_deficit_hyperactivity_disorder

94. Crichton, A. (1798). *An inquiry into the nature and origin of mental derangement: Comprehending a concise system of the physiology and pathology of the human mind: History of the passions and their effects.* Vol 1. T. Cadell, Junior, and W. Davies. Retrieved 19 June 2013.

95. History of attention deficit hyperactivity disorder. (n.d.) *en.wikipedia.org.* Retrieved from http://en.wikipedia.org/wiki/History_of_attention_ deficit_hyperactivity_disorder

96. Diagnostic and Statistical Manual of Mental Disorders. (n.d.) *psychiatry. org.* Retrieved from https://www.psychiatry.org/psychiatrists/practice/ dsm, p. 79.

97. Hinshaw, S.P., & Scheffler, R.M. (2014). p. 20.

98. Attention deficit hyperactivity disorder: Causes of ADHD. (May 1, 2017). *webmd.com.* Retrieved from http://www.webmd.com/add-adhd/guide/adhd-causes

99. Barkley, R. (May 4, 2000). Medicating kids. Interview Frontline PBS. *pbs.org.* Retrieved from http://www.pbs.org/wgbh/pages/frontline/ shows/medicating/interviews/barkley.html

100. Low, K. Causes of attention-deficit/hyperactivity disorder. (May 30, 2017). *verywell.com.* Retrieved from http://add.about.com/od/adhdthebasics/a/ causes.htm

101. Koch, K. What causes ADHD? 12 myths and facts (n.d.). *health.com.* Retrieved from http://www.health.com/health/gallery/0,,20441463,00. html

102. Hinshaw, S.P., & Scheffler, R.M. (2014), p. 22.

103. Understanding ADHD. (n.d.) *chadd.org*. Retrieved from http://www. chadd.org/Understanding-ADHD/TheDisorderNamedADHDWWK1. aspx.

104. What causes ADHD? (n.d.) *attitudemag.com*. Retrieved from http:// www.additudemag.com/adhdblogs/19/8209.html

105. Hinshaw & Scheffler. (2014). pp. xii–xiv

106. Barkley, R. (May 4, 2000).

107. About ADHD. (n.d.) *chadd.org* Retrieved from http://www.chadd.org/ Understanding-ADHD/About-ADHD.aspx

108. Ballas, Paul (2 April 2008). ADHD dynamic history: The effects of continuously changing diagnostic criteria. *Health Central*. Remedy Health Media. Retrieved from https://www.healthcentral.com/article/adhds-dynamic-history-the-effects-of-continuously-changing-diagnostic-criteria

109. Barkley, R.A. (2006). *Attention deficit hyperactivity disorder: A handbook for diagnosis and treatment* (3rd ed.). New York: Guilford Press.

110. Lange, K.W, Reichl, S., Lange, K.M., Tucha, L., & Tucha, O. (30 November 2010). "The history of attention deficit hyperactivity disorder". *Attention Deficit Hyperactivity Disorders* 2 (4): 241–55. Retrieved from https://link.springer.com/article/10.1007%2Fs12402-010-0045-8/fulltext.html.

111. Iannelli, V. (March 14, 2011).

112. Alcantara, J. (October 7, 2008). Attention Deficit Hyperactivity Disorder. *icpa4kids.org*. Retrieved from http://icpa4kids.org/Wellness-Articles/ attention-deficit-hyperactivity-disorder.html

113. Ballas, Paul (April 2, 2008). "ADHD's Dynamic History: The Effects of Continuously Changing Diagnostic Criteria". *Health Central*. Remedy Health Media.

114. Strauss A.A., & Lehtinen, L.E. (1947). *Psychopathology and education of the brain-injured child*. New York: Grune & Stratton.

115. Strauss, A.A., & Kephart, N.C. (1955). *Psychopathology and education of the brain-injured child. Volume II. Progress in theory and clinic*. New York: Grune & Stratton.

116. Lange, Klaus W., (30 November 2010).

117. Heward, W.L. (July 20, 2010). http://www.education.com/partner/articles/pearson/ Causes of learning disability. education.com Retrieved from: http://www.education.com/reference/article/causes-learning-disabilities.

118. Schrag, P., & Divoky, D. (1975), (p. 47). See also: Hobbs, N. (December 15, 1973.) "The Futures of Children; Categories, Labels and Their Consequences," report of the Project on Classification of Exceptional Children. https://eric.ed.gov/?id=ED115069.

119. Schrag, P., & Divoky, D. (1975). *The myth of the hyperactive child & other means of child control*. (pp. 48–50). New York: Pantheon Books.

120. Heward, W. L. (July 20, 2010)

121. Kohn, A. (1989). Suffer the restless children. *Atlantic Monthly*, 95–96.

122. Holliman, R., & Koehler, C. (n.d.) Mental health detectives: Getting to the bottom of diagnosing ADHD. *txca.org*. Retrieved from https://www.txca.org/images/tca/Documents/Conference/PGC13/Handouts/118.pdf

123. Brown, T. (n.d.) ADHD brain scans: Are these necessary for a diagnosis? *attitudemag.com*. Retrieved from https://www.additudemag.com/adhd-brain-scan-is-it-necessary-to-diagnose

124. Kohn, A. (1989). Suffer the restless children. *Atlantic Monthly*, 95–96.

125. Holliman, R., & Koehler, C. (n.d.)

126. Corkum P.V., Siegel L.S. (1993). Is the continuous performance task a valuable research tool for use with children with attention-deficit-hyperactivity disorder? *J Child Psychol Psychiatry*. 1993; 34:1217–1239. [PubMed]

127. Shaw, P., Eckstrand, K., Sharp, W., Blumenthal, J., Lerch, J.P., Greenstein, D., ... Rappoport, J.L. (2007). Attention-deficit/hyperactivity disorder is characterized by a delay in cortical maturation. Proceedings of the National Academy of Sciences of the United States of America, 104, 19649–19654.

128. The teenage brain: How do we measure maturity? (n.d.) *psychologicalscience.org*. http://www.psychologicalscience.org/news/were-only-human/the-teenage-brain-how-do-we-measure-maturity.html#.WMGroxiZOl4

129. Sowell, E.R., Thompson, P.M., & Holmes C.J., et al. (1999). In vivo evidence for post-adolescent brain maturation in frontal and striatal regions. *Nature Neurosci*. 1999; 2:859–861.

130. Johnson, S., Blum, R., & Giedd, J. (September 2009). Adolescent Maturity and the Brain: The Promise and Pitfalls of Neuroscience Research in Adolescent Health Policy *ncbi.nlm.nih.gov*. Retrieved from https://www.ncbi.nlm.nih.gov/pmc/articles/PMC2892678/

131. Bush, G. (2010). Attention-deficit/hyperactivity disorder and attention networks. *Neuropsychopharmacology*, *35*, (1), 278–300; Bush, G. (2011). Cingulate, frontal, and parietal cortical dysfunction in attention-deficit/hyperactivity disorder. *Biological Psychiatry*, *69*(12), 1160–1167.

132. Hinshaw, S.P., & Scheffler, R.M. (2014), p. 30.

133. Block, M. (n.d.)

134. Baughman, F.A. (2002)

135. Buttross, S.L. (2007) *Understanding attention deficit hyperactivity disorder*. (p. 32) Jackson, Mississippi: University Press of Mississippi.

136. Henion, A., & Elder, T. (August 17, 2010).

137. Wender, P.H. (2000). *ADHD: Attention-deficit hyperactivity disorder in children, adolescents, and adults*. New York: Oxford University Press.

138. Medicating Children. (April 2001). *pbs.org*. Retrieved from http://www.pbs.org/wgbh/pages/frontline/shows/medicating/interviews/barkley.html
139. Hinshaw, S.P., & Scheffler, R.M. p. 30.
140. Wender, P.H. (1995). *Attention-deficit hyperactivity disorder in adults.* (p. 20). New York: Oxford University Press
141. Baughman, F.A. (2002).
142. What causes ADHD? (n.d.) *myadhd.com*. Retrieved from http://www.myadhd.com/causesofadhd.html.
143. Attention Deficit Hyperactivity Disorder: Causes of ADHD. (n.d.) *webmd.com*. Retrieved from http://www.webmd.com/add-adhd/guide/adhd-causes#1
144. Hinshaw, S.P., & Scheffler, R.M. (2014), p. 19.
145. Retrieved from http://www.health.com/health/gallery/0,,20441463,00.html
146. Coghill D., & Banaschewski, T. (2009) The genetics of attention-deficit/hyperactivity disorder. Expert Rev. *Neurother.*; 9:1547–1565.
147. Faraone S.V. et al. (2005). Molecular genetics of attention-deficit/hyperactivity disorder. *Biological Psychiatry*, 57: 1313–1323.
148. Barkley, R.A. (1997). *ADHD and the nature of self-control.* (pp. 31–37) New York: Guilford Press.
149. Furman L.M. (July 2008). "Attention-deficit hyperactivity disorder (ADHD): does new research support old concepts?". *J. Child Neurol.* 23 (7): 775–84.
150. Smalley, S.L. "Behavioral Genetics '97—Genetic Influences on *Childhood*-Onset Psychiatric Disorders: Autism and Attention-Deficit/Hyperactivity Disorder," *American Journal of Human Genetics*, vol. 60 (1997), pp. 1276–82.
151. Hinshaw, S.P., & Scheffler, R.M. (2014), p. 28.
152. Pauls, D.L. The Genetics of Attention-Deficit/Hyperactivity Disorder. *Biological Psychiatry*. 2005, Vol 57, issue 11, pp. 1310, 1312.
153. Neale B.M., Medland S., Ripke S., et al. (2010). Case-control genome-wide association study of attention-deficit/hyperactivity disorder. *J Am Acad Child Adolesc Psychiatry* (2010); 49: 906–920.
154. Neale B.M., Medland S.E., Ripke S., et al. (2010). Meta-analysis of genome-wide association studies of attention-deficit/hyperactivity disorder. *J Am Acad Child Adolesc Psychiatry* (2010); 49: 884–897.
155. Wender, P.H. (2000). ADHD: *Attention-deficit/hyperactivity disorder in children, Adolescents and adults.* (p. 49). New York: Oxford University Press, USA.
156. Faraone, S.V., Doyle, A.E., Mick, E., & Biederman, J. (2001). Meta-analysis of the association between the 7-repeat allele of the dopamine D4

receptor gene and attention deficit hyperactivity disorder. *American Journal of Psychiatry,* 158, 1052–1057.

157. Hinshaw, S.P., & Scheffler, R.M. (2014), p. 30.
158. First direct evidence that ADHD is a genetic disorder: Children with ADHD more likely to have missing or duplicated segments of DNA. (September 30, 2010). *Sciencedaily.org.* Retrieved from https://www.sciencedaily.com/releases/2010/09/100929191312.htm
159. Willcutt, E. (*in press*). The etiology of ADHD: Behavioral and Molecular Genetic approaches. In D. Barsch (Ed.), *Cognitive and Affective Neuroscience of Psychopathology.* Oxford University Press. Retrieved from http://psych.colorado.edu/~willcutt/pdfs/Willcutt_ADHD_genetics_inpress.pdf (p. 14)
160. Willcutt, E. p. 14. (Critique: The first possibility—parental responsibility. Excluding the most appalling of situations, parents do not cause a child's school (or home) struggles. That parents inadvertently contribute to the child's behaviors, and thus to the child school-related difficulties, is to add them to the dozen other variables that compose a child's environmental life space. The probability of a gene that contributes to a child's non-compliance, is about the same as catching a falling star. Dr. Thapar's purported findings must stand or fall on their own merit. In the present case, her conclusion that she's discovered a genetic link to ADHD is not correct. Genes *are* measurable, and observable. Genes are link to physiology and chemistry and their behavior manifestations. ADHD has no physiology or chemistry. It's a name.

The second possibility, perinatal screening, rings more of science fiction than fact. One assumes that an evaluation of a child's genotype during the first month of life will reveal the child's genetic code. To suggest that the code will reveal what shortcomings a child will experience in learning, attention, impulse control is neither plausible nor necessary. Parents who watch their child develop during the early months and years will come to know their child's social, cognitive, and behavioral predilections. Alert, informed parents will perceive discrepancies. They will know what questions to ask, and what data to gather (See Strategies.) There's much they can do to assist their child without invading the youngster's genes.

The third possibility is on one hand appalling, and on the other hand difficult to understand. Psychosocial interventions alter a person's behavior, thoughts, emotions, perceptions, relationships, etc. They don't alter compromised neurophysiological mechanisms, that assertion holds even if we assume the presence of such ADHD-related physiological irregularities could be documented, which is highly doubtful. Claiming that genetic verification would provide more and better drugs is expected of individuals who possess the narrowest of perspectives when it comes to children's everyday home and school behavior. So fixed on authenticating the construct ADHD, they overlook that children live in their environment, not in their genes. While genes can and do presuppose, most of what they do in everyday life (with important exceptions, of course) is not irreversible. Genetic researchers without agendas readily share that thinking.

161. Barkley, R.A. (September 1998). Attention-deficit hyperactivity disorder. *Scientific American*, p. 71.
162. Thanks to geneticist Beth Rosen-Sheidley, via personal communication.
163. Faraone, S.V. et al. (2005) Molecular genetics of attention-deficit hyperactivity disorder. *Biological Psychiatry, 57,* (11) pp. 1313–1323.
164. Freitag, C.M., & Retz, W. (2010). Family and twin studies in attention-deficit hyperactivity disorder. In W. Retz & R. Klein (eds): *Attention-Deficit Hyperactivity Disorder (ADHD) in Adults. Key Issues in Mental Health.* Basel, Karger, 2010, vol 176, pp. 38–57. Retrieved from http://www.karger.com/ProdukteDB/Katalogteile/isbn3_8055/_92/_37/KIMH176_02.pdf
165. Thapar, A., Langley, K., O'Donovan, M. and Owen, M. (2006) Refining the attention deficit hyperactivity disorder phenotype for molecular genetic studies. *Molecular Psychiatry* (2006) 11, 714–720. doi:10.1038/sj.mp.4001831; published online May 16, 2006. Retrieved from http://www.nature.com/mp/journal/v11/n8/full/4001831a.html
166. Chi, T.C., & Hinshaw, S.P. (2002). Mother-child relationship of children with ADHD: The role of maternal depressive symptoms and depression-related distortions. *Journal of Abnormal Child Psychology, 30,* 387–400.
167. Sherman, D.K., Iacono, W.G., & McGue, M.K. "Attention-Deficit-Hyperactivity Disorder Dimensions: A Twin Study of Inattention and Impulse-Hyperactivity," *Journal of the American Academy of Child and Adolescent Psychiatry,* vol. 36, (1997), pp. 745–53.
168. Chilcoat, H.D., & Breslau, N. "Does Psychiatric History Bias Mothers' Reports? An Application of a New Analytic Method," *Journal of the American Academy of Child and Adolescent Psychiatry,* vol. 36, (1997), pp. 971–79.
169. Reid, R., & Vasa, S., Vasa, F., et al. (1994). "An Analysis of Teachers' Perceptions of Attention-Deficit Hyperactivity Disorder," *Journal of Research and Development in Education,* vol. 27, (1994), pp. 195–202.
170. Hinshaw, S.P., & Scheffler, R.M. (2014), p. 38.
171. Wolraich, M.L. Hannah, J.N., et al. (1996). "Comparison of Diagnostic Criteria for Attention-Deficit Hyperactivity Disorder in a County-Wide Sample." *Journal of the American Academy of Child and Adolescent Psychiatry,* vol. 35 (1996), pp. 319–24.

172. Thapar A., Harrington R., Ross K., McGuffin P. Does the definition of ADHD affect heritability? *J Am Acad Child Adolesc Psychiatry*. 2000 December; 39(12):1528–1536.

173. Wood, A.C., & Neale, M.C. (2010). Twin Studies and Their Implications for Molecular Genetic Studies: Endophenotypes Integrate Quantitative and Molecular Genetics in ADHD Research. J Am Acad Child Adolesc Psychiatry. 2010 September; 49(9): 874–883. Published online July 31, 2010. doi:10.1016/j.jaac.2010.06.006. Retrieved from http://www.ncbi.nlm.nih.gov/pmc/articles/PMC3148177/

174. Schwarz, A. (October 9, 2012).

175. Biederman, J., Faraone, S.V., et al. (1995). "High Risk for [ADHD] Among Children of Parents with Childhood Onset of the Disorder: A Pilot Study," *American Journal of Psychiatry*, vol. 153 (1995), pp. 431–35.

176. Greven, C.U., Harlaar, N., Dale, P.S., & Plomin, R. (2011). Genetic Overlap between ADHD Symptoms and Reading Is largely Driven by Inattentiveness rather than Hyperactivity-Impulsivity. *J Can Acad Child Adolesc Psychiatry*. Feb 2011; 20(1): 6–14.

177. Coolidge, F.L. Thede, L.L., Stewart, S.E., & Segal, D.L. (2002) The Coolidge personality and neuropsychological Inventory for children (CPNI). *Behavior Modification*. Vol 26, No. 4, p. 558.

178. Coolidge, F.L. (2002). p. 563

179. Willerman L.: Activity level and hyperactivity in twins. Child Dev 1973; 44:288–293.

180. Retrieved from http://www.karger.com/ProdukteDB/Katalogteile/isbn3_8055/_92/_37/KIMH176_02.pdf

181. Banaschewski, T., Becker, K., Scherag, S., Franke, B., & Coghil. D. (2010). Molecular genetics of attention-deficit/hyperactivity disorder: an overview. *European Child and Adolescent Psychiatry*, Vol 19, pp. 237–257.

182. Freitag, C.M., & Retz, W. (2010)

183. Faraone, S.V. et al. (2005) Molecular genetics of attention-deficit/hyperactivity disorder. *Biological Psychiatry*. 57(11):1313–23

184. Smith, A.K., Mick, E., & Faraone, S.V. (2009) Advances in genetic studies of attention-deficit/hyperactivity disorder. *Curr Psychiatry Rep*, Apr; 11(2):143–8.

185. Smith, A.K., Mick, E., & Faraone, S.V. (2009) Advances in genetic studies of attention-deficit/hyperactivity disorder. *Curr Psychiatry Rep*, Apr; 11(2):143–8.

186. Leboyer, M., Belliver, F., Nosten-Bertrand, M., et al. (1998) Psychiatric genetics: search for phenotypes. *Trends in Neurosciences*, 21, 102–105

187. Skuse, D.H. (May 2001). Endophenotypes and child psychiatry. The British Journal of Psychiatry, May 2001, 178 (5) 395–396; doi:10.1192/

bjp.178.5.395. Retrieved from http://bjp.rcpsych.org/content/178/5/395

188. John, B., & Lewis, K.R. (May, 1966). Chromosome variability and geographic distribution of insects. Vol 152. No. 3723. pp. 711–721.

189. Wood, A.C., & Neale, M.C. (2010).

190. Li, D., Sjam, P.C., Owen, M.J., & He, L. (2006). Meta-analysis shows significant association between dopamine system genes and attention-deficit hyperactivity disorder (ADHD). *Human Molecular Genetics, 15:* 2276–2284.

191. Spiegel, A. (November 22, 2010). Siblings Share Genes, but Rarely Personalities. *npr.org.* Retrieved from http://www.npr.org/2010/11/18/131424595/siblings-share-genes-but-rarely-personalities.

192. Wender, P. (2000). p. 46.

193. Wender, P. (2000). p. 48.

194. Goldberg, S. (2007) Genetics: Why children aren't just like their parents. http://www.nytimes.com/2007/09/25/health/25iht-sngenes.1.7631062.html?_r=0

195. Cortese S., Faraone S.V., Sergeant J. 2011.Misunderstandings of the Genetics and Neurobiology of ADHD: Moving Beyond Anachronisms. *Am J Med Genet Part B* 156:513–516.

196. Chromosome 21 (2017). *ghr.nim.nih.gov.* Retrieved from https://ghr.nlm.nih.gov/chromosome/21

197. Down syndrome. (2017) *ghr.nlm.nih.gov.* Retrieved from http://ghr.nlm.nih.gov/condition/down-syndrome.

198. Moffitt, T.E., & Melchior, M. (2007, Jun). Why does the worldwide prevalence of childhood attention deficit hyperactivity disorder matter? *Am J Psychiatry, 164*(6):856–858.

199. Retrieved from http://www.cdc.gov/ncbddd/adhd/diagnosis.html

200. Diller, L.H. (1998). pp. 61–62.

201. Diller, L.H. (1998) p. 195.

202. Sleator E.K., Ullmann R.K. (January 1981). "Can the physician diagnose hyperactivity in the office?" *Pediatrics* 67 (1): 13–7

203. Schwarz, A. (October 9, 2012)

204. Brown, T.E. (2005). *Attention Deficit Disorder: The unfocused mind in children and adults.* (p. 189) New Haven: Yale University Press. (Tom Brown is Asst. Clinical Professor of Psychiatry at the Yale University School of Medicine; Associate Director of the Yale Clinic for Attention and Related Disorders.)

205. Kohn, A. (1989), pp. 90–96.

206. Breggin, P.R. (1998) *Talking back to Ritalin.* (p. 145). Monroe ME: Common Courage Press. See also: Mayes, S.D., & Bixler, O.E. (1993). Reliability of global impressions for assessing methylphenidate effects in

children with attention-deficit hyperactivity disorder. Perceptual and Motor Skills, 77, 1215–1218

207. Diller, L.H. (1998), pp. 61–62.

208. Brown, T.E. (2005), p. 192.

209. Mota, V.L. and Schachar, R.J. (2000). "Reformulating Attention-Deficit/Hyperactivity Disorder According to Signal Detection Theory," *Journal of the American Academy of Child and Adolescent Psychiatry* 39(9): 1144–1151.

210. Olivera, M. 05/23/2013, *NBCLatino.* See: http://nbclatino. com/2013/05/23/attention-deficit-hyperactivity-disorder-how-many-children-are-misdiagnosed/.

211. Hinshaw, S.P., & Scheffler, R.M. (2014), p. 101.

212. Elder, T.E. (2010). The importance of relative standards in ADHD diagnoses: Evidence based on exact birth dates. *Journal of Health Economics,* 29 (5), 641–656.

213. Symptoms and diagnosis. (n.d.). *cdc.gov.* Retrieved from http://www. cdc.gov/ncbddd/adhd/diagnosis.html

214. Hinshaw, S.P., & Scheffler, R.M. (2014), p. 37.

215. Belliveau, J. (July 14, 2016). ADHD rating scales: What you need to know. *healthline.com.* Retrieved from http://www.healthline.com/ health-slideshow/adhd-rating-scale#3

216. Conners parent questionnaire. (n.d.) *ibergmanmd.com.* Retrieved from http://www.ibergmanmd.com/uploads/3/0/9/3/3093942/parent.pdf

217. Hinshaw, S.P., & Scheffler, R.M. (2014), p. 35.

218. Barkley, R. (1998). *Attention deficit hyperactivity disorder: A handbook for diagnosis and treatment.* (p. 73). New York: Guilford.

219. Degrandpre, R. (1999), p. 132.

220. Freitag, C.M., & Retz, W. (2010).

221. Diller, L.H. (1998), p. 58.

222. 7 common neuromyths that many educators believe. (n.d.) *spring.org.uk.* Retrieved from http://www.spring.org.uk/2014/10/7-common-neuromyths-that-many-educators-believe.php

223. Kohn, A. (November 1989). Suffer the restless children. *theatlantic.com.* Retrieved from http://www.theatlantic.com/magazine/archive/1989/ 11/suffer-the-restless-children/306473/

224. Breggin, P.R. (1998). Psycho-Stimulant Effects on Children: A Primer for School Psychologists and Counselors. *ablechild.org.* Retrieved from http://ablechild.org/resources/important-reading/documents-reports/psycho-stimulant-effects-on-children/. See also: Armstrong, T. (1999) *ADD/ADHD alternatives in the classroom.* Alexandria, VA: Association for Supervision and Curriculum Development. www.ascd.org.

225. Armstrong, T. (1995). *The myth of the ADD child.* New York: Dutton Press.

226. Breggin, P.R., & Breggin, G.R. (1995). The Hazards of Treating "Attention-Deficit/Hyperactivity Disorder" with Methylphenidate (Ritalin). The Journal of College Student Psychotherapy, Vol. 10(2) 1995, pp. 55–72. Retrieved from http://breggin.com/the-hazards-of-treating-adhd-with-ritalin/.

227. The hazards of treating A.D.H.D. with Methylphenidate (Ritalin). *oikos.org.* Retrieved from http://www.oikos.org/deareport.htm

228. Diller, L.H. (1998), p. 54.

229. Diller, L.H. (1998), p. 62.

230. Palmeri, S. (1996).

231. Diller, L.H. (1998), p. 47.

232. Diller, L.H. (1998), p. 61.

233. DeGrandepre, R. (1999). Ritalin Nation. New York: W.W. Norton & Company.

234. Diller, L.H. (1998), p. 63.

235. Hinshaw & Scheffler. (2014). pp. xii–xiv.

236. Understanding ADHD. (n.d.) *chadd.org.* Retrieved from http://www.chadd.org/Understanding-ADHD/TheDisorderNamedADHDWWK1.aspx

237. Lane, C. (May 4, 2014). The NIMH withdraws support for DSM-5. *psychologytoday.com.* Retrieved from https://www.psychologytoday.com/blog/side-effects/201305/the-nimh-withdraws-support-dsm-5. See also: Allen Frances (May 17, 2013). "The New Crisis in Confidence in Psychiatric Diagnosis". *Annals of Internal Medicine.*; Dalal P.K., Sivakumar T. (2009) Moving towards ICD-11 and DSM-5: Concept and evolution of psychiatric classification. Indian Journal of Psychiatry, Volume 51, Issue 4, pp. 310–319; Kendell, R., Jablensky, A (January 2003). "Distinguishing between the Validity and Utility of Psychiatric Diagnoses". *American Journal of Psychiatry* 160 (1): 4–12. doi:10.1176/appi.ajp.160.1.4. PMID 12505793; Baca-Garcia, E., Perez-Rodriguez, M.M., Basurte-Villamor, I., Del Moral, A.L.F., Jimenez-Arriero, M.A., De Rivera, J.L.G., Saiz-Ruiz, J., Oquendo, M.A. (March 2007). "Diagnostic stability of psychiatric disorders in clinical practice". *The British Journal of Psychiatry* 190 (3): 210–216. doi:10.1192/bjp.bp.106.024026. PMID 17329740

238. Allen, F. (May 17, 2013). The New Crisis in Confidence in Psychiatric Diagnosis. *medpagetoday.com.* Retrieved from http://www.medpagetoday.com/upload/2013/5/17/0000605-201308060-00655-1.pdf

239. Allen, F. (May 17, 2013).

240. Greenberg, Gary (January 29, 2012). "The D.S.M.'s Troubled Revision". *The New York Times.*

241. Jabr, F. (January 28, 2013). The newest edition of Psychiatry's "bible," the DSM-5, is complete. scientificamerican.com. Retrieved from http://www.scientificamerican.com/article/dsm-5-update/

242. Diller, L.H. (1998), p. 60.

243. van Pragg, H.M. (1993). *Make-Believes in psychiatry, or the Perils of Progress.* (p. 31). New York: Brunner-Mazel.

244. Allen, F. (May 17, 2013).

245. Dalal P.K., Sivakumar T. (2009) Moving towards ICD-11 and DSM-5: Concept and evolution of psychiatric classification. *Indian Journal of Psychiatry*, Volume 51, Issue 4, pp. 310–319.

246. Thomas Insel, M.D. April 29, 2013. Transforming diagnosis. *nimh.nih. gov.* Retrieved from http://www.nimh.nih.gov/about/director/2013/transforming-diagnosis.shtml.

247. Lane, C. (May 4, 2014).

248. Hinshaw, S.P., & Scheffler, R.M. (2014), p. xxv.

249. Diller, L.H. (1998), p. 14.

250. Schwarz, A. (Oct 9, 2012)

251. Pelham, Jr. W. E. (2005). Medication combined with behavior therapy works best for ADHD children, study finds. sciencedaily.com. Retrieved from https://www.sciencedaily.com/releases/2005/05/050506155008.htm

252. Panksepp, J. (1998). *Affective Neuroscience: the foundations of human and animal emotions.* New York: Oxford University Press. p. 1.

253. Brown, T.E. (2005), p. 313.

254. Rudgley, R. (1993). The alchemy of culture: Intoxicants in society. London: British Museum Press.

255. 5-Hour energy start-up story. Retrieved from https://www.fundable.com/learn/startup-stories/5-hour-energy.

256. http://www.foodnavigator-usa.com/Suppliers2/5-Hour-Energy-ramps-up-from-seven-to-nine-million-bottles-a-week

257. Donald A. Redelmeier, Lorraine E. Ferris, Jack V. Tu, Janet E. Hux, and Michael J. Schull. Problems for clinical judgement: introducing cognitive psychology as one more basic science. *CMAJ.* Feb 6, 2001; 164(3): 358–360.

258. Nisbett R.E., & Ross L. (1980) *Human inference: strategies and shortcomings of social judgment.* (pp. 167–192). Englewood Cliffs (NJ): Prentice Hall; 1980.

259. Diller, L. H. (1998), p. 62.

260. Images in Psychiatry: Charles Bradely, MD. (July 1, 1998). *American Journal of Psychiatry*, Volume 155, Issue 7, July 1998, pp. 968. https://doi.org/10.1176/ajp.155.7.968

261. Mayes, R., & Rafalovich, A. "Suffer the Restless Children: The Evolution of ADHD and Pediatric Stimulant Use," *History of Psychiatry* (Volume

18, No. 4, December 2007: 435–457). Retrieved from http://hpy.sage-pub.com/cgi/content/abstract/18/4/435

262. Sroufe, L.A. (January 28, 2012). Ritalin Gone Wrong. *nytimes.com*. Retrieved from http://www.nytimes.com/2012/01/29/opinion/sun-day/childrens-add-drugs-dont-work-long-term.html?_r=0

263. Weiss, G., Minde, K., Douglas, V., Werry, J., & Sykes, D. Comparison of the effects of Chlorpromazine, Dextroamphetamine and Methylphenidate on the Behaviour and Intellectual Functioning of Hyperactive Children, *Canadian Medical Association Journal, 104*, (1971), pp. 20–25.

264. Sroufe, L.A. (January 28, 2012).

265. Rapoport, J.L. (1978). Dextroamphetamine: Cognitive and behavioral effects in normal prepubertal boys. *Science, 199* (4328), 560–563; Rapoport, J.L. (1980). Dextroamphetamine: Its cognitive and behavioral effects in normal and hyperactive boys and normal men. *Archives of General Psychiatry, 37*(8), 933–943.

266. *Neuropsychopharmacology* (2006) 31, 2376–2383. doi:10.1038/sj.npp.1301164; published online July 19 July 2006.

267. Baughman, F.A. See: http://psychrights.org/research/Digest/ADHD/ADHDAsFraud.ht

268. DeGrandpre, R. (1999).

269. Diller, L.H. (1998), p. 314.

270. https://www.washingtonpost.com/national/health-science/still-more-questions-than-answers-about-how-to-treat-adhd/2015/06/01/294b0df2-c738-11e4-aa1a-86135599fb0f_story.html?utm_term=.9f72e3bfbd5f

271. Peloquin, L., & Klorman, R. (1986). Effects of methylphenidate on nor-mal children's moods, event-related potentials, and performance in mem-ory, scanning and vigilance. *Journal of Abnormal Psychology, 95*, 88–98.

272. http://www.kevinmd.com/blog/2013/12/movement-decon-struct-adhd-diagnosis.html

273. Jacobs, B. ADD & ADHD – Epidemic of a phantom disease. Extracted from *Nexus Magazine*, Volume 12, Number 2 (February–March 2005) Retrieved from https://www.nexusmagazine.com/products/down-loads/individual-articles-downloads/volume-12-article-downloads/vol-12-no-2-downloads/add-adhd-epidemic-of-a-phantom-disease-detail.

274. Gualtieri C.T., Johnson L.G., & Benedict K.B. (2004). Differentiating between MCI and early dementia with a new, computerized neurocogni-tive screening battery. DOI: 10.1016/j.jalz.2005.06.365

275. Bart, S. (February 8, 2012). Why we should eliminate the diagnosis of ADHD. *Conditions*. See http://www.kevinmd.com/blog/2012/02/eliminate-diagnosis-adhd.html

276. Hallowell, E.M. & Ratey, J.J. (1995). *Driven to distraction*. New York: Pantheon. p. 41 See also: DeGrandpre, R. (1999), (p. 131).
277. Putnam, F.W. (1990). Foreword. In Donovan, D.M. and McIntyre. D. *Healing the hurt child*. New York: W.W. Norton. See also: Breggin, P. R. (1998) *Talking back to Ritalin*. (p.186). Monroe ME: Common Courage Press.
278. Hinshaw, S.P. & Scheffler, R.S. "Expand Pre-K, Not A.D.H.D." February 23, 2014, *New York Times*.
279. Henion, A., & Elder, T. (August 17, 2010)
280. Furman, L. (2005). What is Attention Deficit Hyperactivity Disorder (ADHD? *Journal of Child Neurology*, 20, 994–1002.
281. Jacobs, B. (February-March 2005).
282. Gualtieri C.T., Johnson L.G., & Benedict K.B. (2004).
283. Forbes G.B. Clinical utility of the test of variables of attention (TOVA) in the diagnosis of attention-deficit/hyperactivity disorder. *Journal of Clinical Psychology*. 1998; 54:461–76. [PubMed].
284. Diller, L.H., (1998), p. 319.
285. Groopman, J. (2008) *How Doctors Think*. Boston: Houghton Mifflin Harcourt.
286. Breggin, P. (October 13, 2011) A.D.H.D. Is a Misdiagnosis. *nytimes.com*. Retrieved from https://www.nytimes.com/roomfordebate/2011/10/12/are-americans-more-prone-to-adhd/adhd-is-a-misdiagnosis
287. Schwarz, A. (November 14, 2014) One Drug or 2? Parents See Risk but Also Hope. *nytimes.com*. Retrieved from http://www.nytimes.com/2014/11/15/us/one-drug-or-2-parents-see-risk-but-also-hope.html?_r=0.
288. Elia J., Borcherding B.G., Rapoport J.L., Keysor C.S. Methylphenidate and dextroamphetamine treatments of hyperactivity: Are there true non-responders? *Psychiatry Res*. 1991; 36:141–155. [PubMed].
289. Schwarz, A. (Oct 9, 2012).
290. Johnson, R.A., Kenney, J.B., & Davis, J.B. Journal: *The School Review, vol. 85*,(1976) no. 1, pp. 91–92; Lennard, H., Epstein, L., Bernstein, A., and Ransom, D. "Hazards implicit in prescribing psychoactive drugs", *Science*, 169, (1970) pp. 438–41.
291. Miller, C. (n.d.) What We Know about the Long-Term Effects of ADHD Medications and What We Don't Know. *childmind.org*. Retrieved from https://childmind.org/article/know-long-term-effects-adhd-medications/.
292. Robitti, S. (August 15, 2014). Long-Term Effects of Drugs Used for ADHD. *medshadow.org*. Retrieved from http://medshadow.org/adhd/adhd-resources/.

293. Dobson, W. (n.d.) ADHD Medications: Are There Any Long-Term Side Effects, Risks? *Additudemag.com*. Retrieved from http://www.additudemag.com/adhdblogs/19/12089.html.

294. Reuters. (May 5, 2014).

295. Berman, S., Kuczenski, R., McCracken, J.T., & London, E.D. (2009). Potential Adverse Effects of Amphetamine Treatment on Brain and Behavior: A Review. *Mol Psychiatry*. 2009 Feb; 14(2): 123–142. Retrieved from http://www.nature.com/mp/journal/v14/n2/full/mp200890a.html

296. Schwarz, A. (December 14, 2013).

297. Diller, L.H. (1998), p. 116.

298. Attention Deficit Hyperactivity Disorder. (n.d.) *nimh.nih.gov*. Retrieved from https://www.nimh.nih.gov/health/topics/attention-deficit-hyperactivity-disorder-adhd/index.shtml.

299. Attention Deficit Hyperactivity Disorder. (n.d.) *nimh.nih.gov*

300. Attention Deficit Hyperactivity Disorder. (n.d.) *nimh.nih.gov*

301. Robert Whitaker. (2013, March 20). *Medicating ADHD: Diagnosis and the Long-Term Effects of the Medications.* Podcast retrieved from http://www.scienceforthepublic.org/medical-research/medicating-adhd-diagnosis-and-the-long-term-effects-of-the-medications/

302. In Baughman, F.A. (2006) *ADHD Fraud: How psychiatry makes patients of normal children.* (p. 62). Victoria BC: Trafford Publishing.

303. Whalen, C.K., & Hencker, B. (1980) The Social Ecology of Psychostimulant Treatment: A Model for Conceptual and Empirical Analysis. In C.K. Whalen & B. Hencker (Eds.) *Hyperactive Children: The social ecology of identification and treatment.* New York: Academic Press.

304. Diller, L.H. (1998), p. 330.

305. Frances, A. (April 2, 2014) Commentary: Treat the Classroom, Not the Kids. *Psychiatric Times.*

306. Braaten, E. (March 2016). Are increased academic demands causing ADHD? mghclaycenter.org. Retrieved from http://www.mghclaycenter.org/parenting-concerns/pre-school/are-increased-academic-demands-causing-adhd/

307. DeGrandpre, R. (1999).

CHAPTER 5

Active Intervention

Professor Emeritus James M. Kauffman's wise counsel reminds us:

[O]ur job as educators (especially, as special educators) is to try to figure out what differences are most important for teaching. As far as I can figure out to date, the differences we need to be most concerned about—maybe the only ones—are (a) what the student knows about whatever we're trying to teach and (b) what that student needs to learn next about whatever we're trying to teach. Then we need to find out how to teach that next thing most effectively and efficiently. And I think this is true regardless of any other differences that we may know exist, many, most, or all of which may be irrelevant to the task of teaching.[1]

We've lost Dr. Kauffman's unpretentious perspective on many occasions. Rather than intervene actively on behalf of an academically struggling child, rather than determine "what the student knows about whatever we're trying to teach," we go on a hunt for a categorical name and its implied explanation as if without either there's little we can do to assist the youngster. It's an acquired obsession, or one that's forced upon us by state and/or federal regulations. Why this continued, curious pursuit while the child slips deeper into the hole that we've helped create? We've already covered one reason for this quest: the belief that the name will tell us what to do. That thinking has been shown to be faulty. Consider the diagnostic categories that neurologist Martin Kutscher lists for us in his book, "Kids In The Syndrome Mix…"[2]

© The Author(s) 2017
J. Macht, *The Medicalization of America's Schools*,
DOI 10.1007/978-3-319-62974-2_5

- ADHD LD autism spectrum (ASD);
- obsessive-compulsive disorder (OCD);
- Tourette's syndrome; Bipolar disorder;
- oppositional defiant disorder (ODD);
- Central auditory processing disorder; and,
- Sensory-motor integration dysfunction, to which I will add Dyslexia Dysgraphia Dyscalculia
- Intellectual and Developmental Disabilities (IDD)
- emotionally disturbed (ED)
- mild mental retardation (MMR).

Despite their authoritative-sounding names, none of the classifications provide anything of practical *strategic* value. They are properly umbrellas, constructs that need to be used as adjectives to describe a child, and never used as nouns to explain the child's observable, often troubling, behavior. Strange, though, that regardless of how the terms are used, by themselves they are empty, tautological distractions. To build effective strategies designed to help a struggling school child we need to discover each youngster's educational, emotional, environmental, and intellectual strengths to build the best-fit intervention. We discover such by careful assessments and analyses, both accomplished by observing the child's actions within context. Construct names like the above provide none of that. More egregious, of course, would be to designate a child "disabled" and conclude further that the above presumed disabilities explain a child's educational underachievement or counterproductive behavior. That improper perspective overlooks the essential contributing variables that are actively influencing the youngster, again, what can only be found by examining closely how the child fits within his/her environmental context both at school and home. Such listed categorical demarcations serve administrative needs, both federal and state governmental agencies that oversee schools and their practices. The labels do little to improve a child's circumstance. Indeed, the contrary might be the case. By accepting any one of the listed "conditions" as causative, we often look no further for contributing variables, a major oversight on our part.

Diagnosis of the apparent reasons for under-functioning in children with special needs has a very poor track record in terms of informing special educational practice. The history of special education is littered over recent decades with a plethora of ill conceived and subsequently debunked diagnostic procedures. There has been precious little to show for their effectiveness if you look at the research evidence, in spite of the publicity that many of them continue to attract. We should be aware that in special education, as in so many fields where people feel desperate for help, the door is wide open both for manifest, unabashed, charlatans (with the latest snake oil in their medicine show) and also for the well-meaning, sincere, but just plain wrong-headed, self-appointed "saviours." People whose children have disabilities or learning difficulties are very sensitive and susceptible to the blandishments of those who purport to have the answer but have no research evidence with which to substantiate their claims.[3]

As you know, disability names also factor in to special education's eligibility decisions, specifically which children are provided additional resource assistance. That's another reason we search out "disabilities."

That the children are plainly struggling with their studies, and often their behavior, is, unfortunately, not seen as sufficient grounds to earn timely, intensive, individualized resource assistance. Without a confirmed diagnostic category, LD, for example, no matter its functional irrelevancy, eligibility may not be granted and services may not be provided. (Please see "gatekeeper" below. The effort to disqualify a child from needed services is often intentional.) The outcome sadly is predictable. We often lose a child, both figuratively and literally.

> In one of my classes, there was a young man who approached me after school. He, at seventh grade level, begged me to teach him the alphabet. I could not fathom that anyone who had reached seventh grade did not know the alphabet, but he did not. Being a new teacher, not familiar with any protocols within the school system, I met with his parent, and he was referred for Special Education. I lost track of him, and did not know if he is doing well or if he is even alive. I did get a letter from him after he graduated high school; it was written by his girlfriend because he still could not write. She also struggled with writing.[4] —Sharon Thoner, MS, Special Education Teacher

How is it possible that a young man, with courage and acumen enough to approach a veritable stranger and ask for help, could not know his alphabet by seventh grade? If you answered, "Something must be wrong with the youngster," then you've embraced the medical model. "Q": Allowing for that possibility, and even presuming that the yougster has verifiable brain damage, what do you suppose happens next? "A": Do accountable schools have any solution other than find a willing, well-trained teacher? Exactly what could they have done when someone *first* noticed this young man's difficulty learning the alphabet years earlier? Why was he not provided early services? He might not have qualified. His IQ score (or more aptly, his EQ score) might have been a few points too low, and someone without a lot of smarts presumed the boy's pint jug had reached its maximum capacity. Try to justify that thinking in a court of justice.

There's a third reason we go hunting. It allows us to, euphuistically, move the child along, meaning we let someone else accept responsibility for the youngster and his/her often difficult, irritating ways. I remember more than one occasion where a decidedly challenging child was declared "cured" when he and his parents moved to a different state.

> I am in hell—or its equivalent. Specifically, I am in an IEP meeting [Individual Educational Plan] for my daughter, a special-education student. ... My daughter's reading comprehension and vocabulary skills are ranked as "very superior"; her learning issues center on math. Some teachers assume that a child who is smart in one area is simply being lazy or obstructionist by not being smart in another. After three years at an elementary school with the county's highest standardized test scores where she was constantly told that she "just needed to *focus*," my daughter collapsed to the floor one night sobbing. She'd spent two hours on (math) homework (that might have been done in 30 minutes). ... The school's institutional culture regarded kids with learning disabilities as impediments to their goal of keeping those standardized scores high. The emotional toll exacted on a child who is told that his repeated failures are his own fault can be high.

> An educator sitting close to me says she has a great (new) place for my daughter: a program at one of the county's lower-performing ... schools for kids who have emotional disabilities or autism ... [or], a school for kids with a variety of learning disabilities, where kids' brains are wired differently, [or one] for kids with autism and emotional disabilities; [or], a school [with] kids with dyslexia [and] ADHD.[5]

Imagine how the mom felt when she learned what the school system had in mind for her daughter, who by any reasonable appraisal needed expert help with her mathematics. Instead, Mom was offered: "Let's try a place where she'll get to hang out with children with autism, emotional disturbance, dyslexia, and ADHD." That's more a sign of a problem-shifter than a problem-solver.

Then there's the overzealous professional who takes this categorical naming business to excess, almost like it's a part of a board game that rewards a diagnostician for landing on the most disability squares. Where's our self-governing? Don't you think there's a point of diminishing returns where diagnostic markers completely conceal a child behind our name-calling madness? What is a parent to do with the following but first scream then cry?

I am dealing with my 9-yr. old. He is diagnosed with PDD, NOS, ADHD, ODD, and mood disorder. I also have another child with PDD, NOS, ADHD, and MR. My 9-year old runs the show and I fear my other child … will explode at any moment. My 9-year old has taken: Risperdal, Seroquel, Geodon, and soon his psychiatrist may try Abilify.

Or this:

I have a 10-year old girl, with an always changing diagnoses … she has a bit of everything. Comorbidity of LD, Anxiety, SPD, OCD, ADD, as well as Aspie [Asperger's] traits.[6]

Even the most experienced clinician would need a few deep breaths before saying anything useful or supportive to either parent.

BEYOND NAMES

We need to get beyond these names. They're shackles that bind our thinking. They're forgeries, claiming to be real when they're worthless currency. We don't need them to help any child. They're medical model trivia that say more about the diagnostician than the youngster. Take any one of the above children in their present state, as difficult as it might be. Without one categorical name mentioned, we have all the technology necessary to help the young lady extricate herself (and her parents) from her mathematical nightmare, all the knowledge we need to aid the young man out of his embarrassing plight that's left him unable to write a letter to his girlfriend or his parents, and all the experience necessary to provide the mom and her two boys with options besides a fifth round of medication that's likely doing untold damage to the boys' physiology.

Let's take a case.

Suppose we have a 7-year old youngster who struggles to write his name. If we choose to search out a disability name, which strategically is completely unnecessary, and if we're guided by special education's defunct discrepancy model, which is also completely unnecessary, we'll pull out David Wechsler's "Intelligence test for children," and discover the child scores low on a measure of his IQ. How low? It really doesn't matter, not if we're determined to help the child. It just means a different name, some variation of old school "mental retardation" or "developmental delay," where one construct label is as functionally useless as another. Interestingly, a sharp school psychologist could discover a smattering of a child's strengths and weaknesses from even this misnamed normative test, though s/he'd accomplish much more with a series of non-normative tests, assuming s/he's more interested in learning about the child and what he needs, rather than what categorical name to use on a form.

Or we could decide that an IQ score was a worthless measure, as would be the name designation "Intellectually and developmentally delayed," that the hours involved to make the assessment could be put to much better use. We know what to do. We don't have to wait for anyone's permission. Watch this, please, the purpose less to draw attention to the procedure and more to share that it's available. The procedure combines what's termed "shaping" with "fading," and with "contingencies," what most special education teachers are familiar with, and, collectively, along with good teacher sense, what needs to be a part of all elementary school teachers' professional training.

(**FYI: Shaping** is used when a *target* behavior does not yet exist. In **shaping**, you support or reinforce an *approximation* to the target behavior. "Approximation" means any behavior that resembles the desired behavior or takes the child closer to the desired goal. We'd use shaping to help each of the youngsters mentioned earlier, categorical names not invited. We'd show the children's parents (and teachers, if they're willing to participate) how to use the procedure, which is as much an attitude as a structured strategy.)

Name Writing

A 7-year-old struggled to write the letters of his name, a goal his parents and his teacher had established. His verbal skills were delayed, as were his motor skills. The school psychologist might have spent important time with the parents explaining individual differences and possible factors that produce such intellectual and/or performance differences (not disabilities). To the question why the child is so different from others, the psychologist would have used his/her skills to convince Mom and Dad that what's most important is to help their child grow stronger and more confident academically.

Teacher accounts revealed that the boy had fought the assignment for months: nothing about it was enjoyable; nothing he did was successful. (A self-regulating educator would have realized that the strategies s/he used were ineffective long before the child "struggled for months." As long as we continue to sequester resource personnel, making them available only after a positive eligibility hearing, we'll have large numbers of children who struggle for months, curriculum rigor mortis gaining ground as the unsuccessful days pass. That's hardly a proactive, child-centered system.)

I assigned one of my college students to the child and his teacher. The psychology student reported that the teacher failed to provide the stressed child with either prompts (to be faded) or incentives to spur him on, skills the regular teacher may not have possessed.

Observations revealed the child's entering writing skills. He held the pencil in his closed fist, point down as his writing hand flew in the air rather than resting comfortably on the table. The penciled lines scattered across the paper bore no relationship to any letter. To assist the child, several pencil grips were borrowed from other teachers. The child chose the one he liked best.

The shaping/**fading** steps included:

1. With pencil grasped correctly, the child (with suitable modeling) learned to rest the soft part of the writing hand on the table.
2. The child was provided paper upon which were printed letters composed of printed dots (prompts) rather than solid lines used to enhance tracing. Each set of letter-forming dots were positioned within a small drawn rectangle (prompt) that provide the child structure intended to maintain his attention to letter size and position vis-à-vis subsequent letters of his name. (Analysis suggested the child had a good sense of writing left to right, but not to incorporate left to right in a relatively straight, horizontal line.)
3. As the child learned to connect the dots and thus write the targeted letter, the prompting dots were gradually faded out (from 12 dots per letter to 8 to 6) until one dot served as the starting point still located within the prompting rectangle. Eventually, only the rectangle remained, the space within which the child was to write his letter. Eventually, only the bottom line of the rectangle remained, mirroring a lined piece of paper. Soon, the bottom line was no longer needed as the child learned to write the letters in small spaces without any structure beyond the paper the teacher provided. The child continued to use the pencil grip until he decided he no longer needed its support.

From the beginning of the intervention—with the first step of the shaping procedure well *within* the child's skill set, the youngster was provided time with his favorite Legos when he completed the increasingly complex steps. The child learned that when he completed the letter-writing task the teacher required (the task well defined and explained), he earned his treasured Legos for 1 minute. A sand timer was used to display his reinforcement time.

The incentive was sufficient to encourage the child to try the activity. The task divided into parts enabled the child to experience the incentive early on while gradually learning to connect dots and eventually write, without the prompts, the letters of his name. The process included frequent brief trials, frequent brief reinforcement, and steady acquisition of the skills. With the task no longer unpleasant (and unsuccessful), the child's writing effort required little additional encouragement—though the teacher continued to express her appreciation for the child's hard work—as she did with all her pupils.

With respect to this child, the teacher (and the school staff) might have spent an inordinate amount of professional time and energy designating what's wrong with the child, rather than analyzing his skill sets, seeking to identify the child's precise academic and motor strengths. How he compared to his classmates earned not a moment's thought. From the beginning, we could have done better for the child (meaning we could have helped the child sooner) had we embraced a non-categorical perspective.

"Q" (the following question was presumably raised by a teacher): "Wouldn't it be better to separate students into classes based on certain disability categories? In that way, all students could get the specific help they need." ("Q": Before proceeding further, could you explain to the teacher who asked this question what was wrong with her assumption that "the children would get the specific help they needed if they were grouped by disability?" Hint: Think "entering skills," rather than diagnostic classifications.)

(Response from an National Education Association (NEA) authority.) It just isn't that simple or clear. The categories of disability that describe students' special education learning needs are often far from unambiguous. In addition, many believe that maintaining a strict categorical approach to serving students often results in fragmented programs and services. One of the reasons states and districts have typically used categorical systems is to limit students' access to special services, rather than to make special services available according to each individual's need—so the categories have actually served as "gatekeepers" in some instances.[7]

(FYI: Elizabeth Farrell (1870–1932) was an educational pioneer. (With others, she would form the Council of Exceptional Children. By all accounts, she was a progressive with extraordinary insights.) Note several of her most salient proposals: Schools should exclude no child; [schools should avoid] overuse of intelligence tests, and [schools should] be responsible for identifying special needs and providing appropriate services, *not just classifying* [children].[8] (Emphasis mine)

(Kevin Wheldall joins the conversation.) Special education is about ways of optimizing the learning environment for people with special needs and disabilities. The majority of special educators in New South Wales, and indeed in Australia, today favor what is known as "a non-categorical approach" to teaching students with special needs (i.e., students with sensory and/or intellectual disabilities, learning difficulties, and/or behavior disorders). Non-categorical programs, according to the Penguin Macquarie Dictionary of Australian Education (1989), "emphasise the skills the child needs for functioning in society, thus avoiding labelling." Labeling, in turn, is defined as "the practice of classifying people into categories and subsequently ascribing to such person or persons the characteristics of the stereotypic member of that category."

Contemporary special educators favoring a non-categorical approach are committed to the conviction that all children can learn, given effective instruction. The forms of pedagogy we employ, however, are determined not by the nature of the child's disabling condition but by a needs-based appraisal of the student's current level of functioning.[9]

What would Dr. Wheldall's suggestions look like if we were to put them into practice where we'd intervene on behalf of a child while bypassing all talk of disabilities? Consider our young lady and her math struggles. If we considered Dr. Wheldall's "needs-based assessment," the outcome for the young lady would differ significantly from what she experienced. Let's help her, again less because of the specific procedures, but because we could have helped her long before she suffered such terrible consequences. We could have interceded when we first noticed her wrestling with her assignments, assuming we held the proper attitude, ideally a non-categorical, pragmatic approach to providing services. (I'll ask you to be the instructional engineer.)

- The fresh-faced, semi-relaxed young lady sits before you, *wary* (as she should be), but ready to give *you* a try. No pressure on anyone. You're not time-driven, and the young lady's not disabled. She has problems with math assignments that are *beyond* her entering skills, as do most of us. That the young lady was a special education student, as Mother indicated, doesn't tell you much, other than at that school with all their diagnostic labels, you're certain the staff were trained exclusively in the medical model rather than the behavior model.

  Notice the differences between the two models.

  The **medical model** presumes that a child's underachieving, inattentive behavior is caused by some neuro-biogenetic irregularity. It sees the child's behavior as disordered and maladaptive.

  The behavior model presumes that a child's current underachieving and/or inattentive behavior is unintentionally maintained by the youngster's home and school environment, rather than being driven by a neuro-biogenetic flaw. It sees the child's behavior as adaptive, where the child does the best s/he can with his/her current skills, home and school support, and prior experiences.

  The **medical model** uses potent chemistry to change a child's physiology.

  The behavior model changes the way significant adults in the child's school and home environment respond to the child to help him/her acquire alternative behaviors.

  Short of swallowing pills, the **medical model** does not require that a youngster be part of the solution. The **medical model** requires little in the way of active participation by the significant adults. It relies on drugs to solve problems *passively*.

  The **behavior model** requires a child's (and his parents' and teachers') *active* participation where the child learns rules and strategies necessary for long-term success.

- First step of the young lady's program. You need to determine what she can do, what math skills she currently possesses. You always start with what a child knows, what physician Paul S. Carbone, with his wife, shared when speaking of their son with autism: "We have always focused on what our son can do and not what he can't."[10] (The advice fits *all* children, label irrelevant.) You'll determine the young lady's "present performance level (PPL), a measure that tells you the level at which the young lady succeeds with math at or near 100%, where she breezes right through problems of all kinds. Those acquired skills represent the successful starting point, what Dr. Wheldall meant by 'needs-based appraisal of the student's current level of functioning'."

- By means of simple paper/pencil assessments that cover a wide range of math problems (the assessments known as "criterion-referenced tests"), you've learned what math exercises the young lady can do with ease. No tears, no stomachaches, no self-deprecation, easy breathing, feeling good. You've identified her PPL. Now you push her a little, just a little, slowly. You know she has a history with unattainable math assignments being forced upon her so you proceed carefully. But you do need the young lady to make errors. From errors, you learn strategies. You're going to do an error analysis, find out what she's missing, what's creating confusion, what *her* school teachers failed to teach her. You go inside her head. "Hey, that was a good answer, just not quite right," you say when she produces the wrong solution. You ask: "How did you get the answer? What did your head tell you to do?" "Walk me through the steps you used. Let's find the glitch."

(**FYI A**: The young lady's school selected its curriculum lessons according to a calendar. It's called "calendar-driven curriculum"—one of the major faults inherent in American public education. Many countries do not assign curriculum on the basis of a calendar (or a child's age). We do both. By selecting lesson plans based on a calendar date, teachers communicate to kids: "What you're ready to learn *isn't* important. *I'm* ready to teach this lesson. Let's get to it." **FYI B**: Teachers always have used the school year calendar to make their [curriculum] plans.[11] It's convenient for them, but not effective for all their students.)

You'll need two essential changes to occur if you're to help this young lady. First, you'll need to locate an excellent math teacher, unless that's you. Based on the error analysis, this math teacher will know how to engineer the small (shaping) steps the youngster will need to *gradually* advance along the math-curriculum ladder, step by step. Second, the young lady's original math teacher, in place of stating that the youngster needs to "focus," needs to modify her curriculum to match the young lady's entering skills. It's called individualization or differentiation. It means the teacher needs to *teach* so the pupil can learn. That's what Dr. Wheldall was aiming toward.

We can do it, we know how to. With the right mindset, that is, one that doesn't require we seek a disability label:

> The term learning disability has appeal because it implies a specific neuro-logical condition for which no one can be held particularly responsible. ... There is no implication of neglect, emotional disturbance, or improper train-ing or education, nor does it imply a lack of motivation on the part of the child. ... For cosmetic purposes, it's a nice term to have around. ... Perhaps most important of all in this incriminating catalog, the term LD says *nothing* to a teacher about how to go about helping a child with his problems.[12] (Emphasis mine)

Taught by staff that held the proper attitude and skills, the young lady's horrific plight could have been completely avoided. That it wasn't avoided, but instead exacerbated, is an indictment against the school that either doesn't know how to regulate itself, or for self-serving reasons, chooses not to regulate itself. Either is unacceptable. It doesn't have to be this way.

A Proper Mindset

> "In physical medicine, physicians look for bacterium that can be identified. If found, medication can be prescribed to combat the bacterium. No such marker exists for ADD. ... To make the diagnosis of ADHD, a clinician must lean heavily on a child's [current and past] history—as reported by parents and teachers."[13] Unlike ailments that are identifiable from physical signs and symptoms and other laboratory parameters, the classification of children's mental disorders, and ADHD in particular, depends on a descrip-tion of behavior derived from adult observations, putting the physician and the parents at a distinct disadvantage. It's accepted that this absence of a definite diagnostic test for [ADHD] not only engenders diagnostic uncer-tainty,[14] it makes the evaluation of information from parents and teachers all the more imperative—though the time-consuming data gathering is often skipped by physicians due to time constraints and overt pressure for a deci-sion from parents.[15]

> Fads in psychiatric diagnosis come and go and have been with us as long as there has been a psychiatry. The fads meet a deeply felt need to explain, or at least to label. Fads punctuate what has become a basic background of overdiagnosis. Normality is an endangered species. It is too bad that there is no advocacy group for normality that could effectively push back against all the forces aligned to expand the reach of mental disorders.[16]

"I had assumed that the Diagnostic and Statistical Manual of Mental Disorders (DSM) leadership used science as a top priority in their decisions. I was told by the head of DSM-IV ... that science was a low priority, and the results of science could be and would be ignored if they conflicted with whatever the DSM leadership wanted to do."[17]

It has long been argued that [the current] system of classifications makes unjustified categorical distinctions between disorders, and uses arbitrary cutoffs between normal and abnormal. [A]ttempts to demonstrate natural boundaries ... have failed.[18]

A valid classification scheme has several essential characteristics. First, it must be possible to measure reliably the individual symptoms which comprise the diagnostic category. It is unlikely that a diagnosis can be reliable, valid, and clinically useful if ... clinicians cannot agree on the definition and measurement of individual symptoms. Second, symptoms should cluster into meaningful syndromes in a consistent manner. Third, the diagnostic entity must be reliable. There is little point in a classification scheme [such as ADHD] that includes categories that cannot be applied in a consistent way by the majority of clinicians and scientists across clinical settings.[19] (Russell Schachar, MD, University of Toronto, Department of Psychiatry)

Our classification system is a hindrance. We'll provide more adequate services in less time if we adopt a non-categorical, non-pathological stance with every child. It's a refreshing challenge. We see each child with obvious and subtle complexities provided and acquired during the full length of his or her young life, each doing the best s/he can with personal strengths and experiences. Nothing is gained from the labels LD or attention-deficit hyperactivity disorder (ADHD), dyslexia, or the other named conditions. If they're needed to earn services, so be it. That's a system weakness. It will take a mammoth wave of parental discontent before wholesale changes can be made where we provide (immediate) services to all kids based on needs, not names. Powerful lobbies exist to maintain the status quo, the participants in the game for themselves, not the children or the children's parents. The respective fields of special education and school psychology could initiate change. If they were so inclined. Nothing is likewise gained from speculating that a child has neurological complications. Rarely are such complications verifiable, much less reversible. Each proposed "biological deficit/defect" used to explain a child's difficult behavior becomes an uninformative tautology, and no one's better for it. Within the medical model, the child's biology is all that matters, not the substance of the child, not the child's parents, not the child's teachers, not life as the child knows it.

"Speaking satirically,"[20] pediatrician Daniel L. Zeidner wrote in the 1995 issue of the journal *Pediatrics,*

> [i]t has become increasingly apparent to me ... that a new syndrome exists among adults who teach our school-aged children: Teacher Deficit Disorder, or TDD. I have observed that this diagnosis should be made on the teacher when the following classic signs and symptoms exist among one or more of his/her students: students who fidget in class, ... who do not pay attention, who frequently daydream, who do not complete their homework or class-work, and who frequently get out of their seats. When students exhibit these manifestations, the teacher should be diagnosed with TDD and, of course, should be medicated immediately with amphetamine or other drugs that should speed him/her up, thus making him/her ... more dynamic and interesting to his/her students.[21]

- We know that schools contribute to the behaviors a clinician uses to designate a child disordered.
- We know that teachers contribute to the behaviors a clinician uses to designate a child disordered.
- We know that schools, their procedures, infrastructure, and instructional demands influence the numbers of children said to have ADHD, LD, dyslexia, and other convenient educational disorders. Achievement and behavioral variability are directly "related to school policies linked to demands for achievement and performance,"[22] demands that often do not match children's preparation and readiness, a direct reference to a "curriculum mismatch."

Maggie Koerth-Baker reported in the *New York Times* that

> Many sociologists and neuroscientists today believe ... that the explosion in rates of diagnosis is caused by sociological factors—especially ones related to education and the changing expectations we have for kids. ... [The] American childhood [has] drastically changed. Even at the grade-school level, kids now have more homework, less recess and a lot less unstructured free time to relax and play. It's easy to look at that situation and speculate how "A.D.H.D." might have become a convenient societal answer for what happens when kids

are expected to be miniature adults. High-stakes standardized testing, increased competition for slots in top colleges, a less-and-less accommodating economy for those who don't get into colleges but can no longer depend on the existence of blue-collar jobs—all of these are expressed through policy changes and cultural expectations, but they may also manifest themselves in more troubling ways—in the rising number of kids whose behavior has become pathologized,[23] [and the children who've become medicalized].

We live in a world that is highly competitive, an intense world that greets our children from the first days of kindergarten. Look at their curriculum; look at what we ask them to do; look at the pressures their parents find themselves facing. There's a must-succeed mentality that places great strain on patience, understanding, differences, and deviations, and being as good as someone else. It's prime for the medical model: it's a fabricated petri dish where discrepancies grow with amazing speed, some much so that medical doctors are ready to medicate three year olds for what amounts to a contrived condition.[24]

The following is a recent Facebook posting that went viral, written by a teacher, Dr. Wendy Bradshaw, who resigned from what she loved to do—teach kids. It says what needs to be said: that schools contribute to the behavior of children, and that we increasingly medicate these children leaving what contributes to their problems *unchanged*.

The children don't only cry. Some misbehave so that they will be the "bad kid" not the "stupid kid", or because their little bodies just can't sit quietly anymore, or because they don't know the social rules of school and there is no time to teach them. My master's degree work focused on behavior disorders, so I can say with confidence that it is not the children who are disordered. The disorder is in the system which requires them to attempt curriculum and demonstrate behaviors far beyond [their readiness skills]. The disorder is in the system which bars teachers from differentiating instruction meaningfully, which threatens disciplinary action if they decide their students need a five-minute break from a difficult concept, or to extend a lesson which is exceptionally engaging. The disorder is in a system which has decided that students and teachers must be regimented to the minute and punished if they deviate. The disorder is in the system which values the scores on wildly inappropriate assessments more than teaching students in a meaningful and research based manner.[25]

NOTES

1. Personal communication from James Kauffman, December 1, 2014.
2. Kutscher, M. L., Attwood, T., & Wolff, R. R. (2014). Kids in the syndrome mix of ADHD, LD, autism spectrum, Tourette's, anxiety and more! London: Jessica Kingsley.
3. Wheldall, K. (1994). Why do contemporary special educators favour (sic) a noncategorical approach to teaching? *musec_contemporary_special_educator.pdf* Retrieved from musec.mq.edu.au/public/download.jsp?id=6411.
4. Personal communication.
5. Thompson, T. (January 3, 2016) The Special-Education Charade: Individualized Education Programs, or IEPs, are one of the greatest pitfalls of the country's school system. *theatlantic.com*. Retrieved from https://www.theatlantic.com/education/archive/2016/01/the-charade-of-special-education-programs/421578/.
6. Lisa. (10/01/2013). *circleofmoms.com*. Retrieved from http://www.circleofmoms.com/moms-kids-adhd/am-i-the-only-mom-of-an-adhd-odd-child-who-feels-like-crying-all-the-time-313491/2.
7. NEA 'IDEA Brief' #6. (n.d.). Wouldn't it be better to separate students into classes based on certain disability categories? In that way all students could get the specific help they need. *nea.org*. Retrieved from http://www.nea.org/home/18719.htm.
8. Duchan, J. (2011). Elizabeth Farrell. *Ascu.buffalo.edu*. Retrieved from http://www.acsu.buffalo.edu/~duchan/new_history/hist19c/subpages/farrell.html.
9. Wheldall, K. (1994).
10. Rosenblatt, A.I., & Carbone, P.S. (2013). *Autism spectrum disorders: What every parent needs to know.* Elk Grove, IL: American Academy of Pediatrics.
11. Jacobs, H.H. (n.d.) Mapping the big picture. *ascd.org*. Retrieved from http://www.ascd.org/publications/books/197135/chapters/The_Need_for_Calendar-Based_Curriculum_Mapping.aspx.
12. Hobbs, Nicholas (1975). The Futures of Children: Categories, Labels, and Their Consequences. (pp. 79–82) Jossey-Bass: San Francisco, CA.
13. Diller, L.H. (1998) *Running on Ritalin: A physician reflects on children, society, and performance in a pill.* (p. 62) New York: Bantam.
14. Zarin, D.A. and Earls, F. (1993) Diagnostic decision making in psychiatry. *American Journal of Psychiatry*, 150, 197–206. See also: Sandberg, Seija. (2002). Hyperactivity and Attention Disorders of Childhood, West Nyack, NY: Cambridge University Press.

15. Schwarz, A., & Cohen, S. (2013). A.D.H.D. Seen in 11% of U.S. Children as Diagnoses Rise. *nytimes.com*. Retrieved from http://www.nytimes.com/2013/04/01/health/more-diagnoses-of-hyperactivity-causing-concern.html?pagewanted%253Dall&_r=0.
16. Frances, A (n.d.) DSM 5 in distress. *psychologytoday.com*. Retrieved from https://www.psychologytoday.com/blog/dsm5-in-distress.
17. Ghaemi, N. (n.d.) Mood swings: a psychiatrist surveys the mind and the wider world. *psychologytoday.com*. Retrieved from https://www.psychologytoday.com/blog/mood-swings/201305/nimh-requiem-dsm-and-its-critics%29--Nassir?page=2.
18. P.K., Sivakumar T. (2009). Moving towards ICD-11 and DSM-5: Concept and evolution of psychiatric classification. Indian Journal of Psychiatry, Volume 51, Issue 4, pp. 310–319.
19. Sandberg, S. (2002). *Hyperactivity and Attention Disorders of Childhood*. West Nyack, New York: Cambridge University Press.
20. Diller, L. (1998). p. 64. *indianjpsychiatry.org*. Retrieved from http://www.indianjpsychiatry.org/article.asp?issn=0019-5545;year=2009;volume=51;issue=4;spage=310;epage=319;aulast=Dalal.
21. Zeidner, D.L. (1995). "Teacher Deficit Disorder". *Pediatrics*, vol. 96, p. 378.
22. Hinshaw, S.P. & Scheffler, R.M. (2014). p. xxv.
23. Koerth-Baker, M. (2013). The not-so-hidden cause behind the A.D.H.D. epidemic. *nytimes.com*. Retrieved from http://www.nytimes.com/2013/10/20/magazine/the-not-so-hidden-cause-behind-the-adhd-epidemic.html?pagewanted=3&_r=2.
24. DeGrandpre, R. (1999). *Ritalin Nation: rapid fire culture and the transformation of human consciousness*. New York: Norton & Company.
25. Einenkel, W. (2015). Teacher's Facebook resignation post goes viral because she is 100% right. *Kosmediallc*. Retrieved from http://www.dailykos.com/story/2015/11/05/1445148/-Teacher-s-Facebook-resignation-post-goes-viral-because-she-is-100-right?detail=email#.

CHAPTER 6

Diversity and the Common Core

The question of who started Common Core is not our concern (Box 6.1).

Box 6.1 Common Core		
Contributor	*Outcome*	*Convenient construct*
Common Core	**Curriculum mismatch**	LD and ADHD-like behaviors

The Internet provides enough options to keep conspiracy theorists busy for hours. The federal government's involvement is not problematic, however, not so much with the standards, but with financial grants provided to states that adopt the movement. States can choose not to adopt the standards, though government's monetary incentives** can make that an unlikely choice for states that need to balance their budgets. (**With any new administration, and any new Secretary of Education, the government's involvement waits to be seen.) Likewise, the movement's stated goals are also not our concern. The goals are honorable: to reverse general education's woes and achieve excellence for *all* US students through the raising of standards and expectations, ensuring those standards

- Reflect "The knowledge and skills that our young people need for success."[1]

© The Author(s) 2017
J. Macht, *The Medicalization of America's Schools*,
DOI 10.1007/978-3-319-62974-2_6

- "Are ... focused on developing critical learning skills instead of mastering fragmented bits of knowledge."
- "Raise expectations for all children, especially those suffering the worse effects of the 'drill and kill' test prep norms of the recent past."[2]

Common Core Standards are currently in place in many schools throughout the USA.[3] The movement has its staunch supporters and its vigorous opponents. As for the children, whether they will benefit from the new standards depends on the individual youngster, how well s/he fits academically within the class of 25 or more kids, and what the child's school holds most important—its state-wide reputation or each child's growth.

If you've never seen a Common Core standard, let's try one. This one pertains to **English Language Arts Standards » Reading: Informational Text** (abbreviated CCSS.ELA-LITERACY.RI.) Many educators believe the standards present themselves as well-orchestrated and challenging, but reasonable and worthwhile. Here's what eight- to nine-year-olds in third grade are expected to do, according to the published standards:

3:1:   Ask and answer questions to demonstrate understanding of a text, referring explicitly to the text as the basis for the answers.
3.2:   Determine the main idea of a text; recount the key details and explain how they support the main idea.
3.3:   Describe the relationship between a series of historical events, scientific ideas or concepts, or steps in technical procedures in a text, using language that pertains to time, sequence, and cause/effect.

"3.1, 3.2, 3.3" represent sequential steps or levels of complexity for third-grade kids—established for every third child, where "every" is the focal word. The child, every child, is expected to accomplish 3.1 before being introduced to 3.2. An *ideal* school system is:

- Where every child's scholastic abilities, positive attitudes, and skill readiness are adequate to the task; and
- Where expert teachers have:
  - time to be creative,
  - time to emphasize, and
  - time to practice,

– time to match curriculum with students, and
– time to move forward and backward within the curriculum sequence.

Common Core and this literacy standard could work quite well with *every* child. At the end of third grade, on paper at least, all kids, whether living in Maine or Honolulu, would demonstrate equal proficiency—on paper, that is. This forecasted outcome is less likely for reasons that will become apparent in just a moment. Before that, understand that Common Core in most elementary schools throughout the USA is not being adopted and applied in settings that reflect much of anyone's ideal. Keep in mind that today's schools are:

• Age-Grade managed, that is, the curriculum is assigned on the basis of age/grade level, not on a child's readiness skills;
• Understaffed;
• Calendar-driven, not performance driven; and
• Replete with highly diverse students whose abilities, skills, and attitudes cover virtually every point on the continuum.

STANDARDS AND DIVERSITY

It's not like Common Core's developers were ignorant of today's pupil diversity and the potential problems resulting from their variable abilities and scattered entering skills. Stated clearly,

> No set of grade-specific standards can fully reflect the great variety of abilities, needs, learning rates, and achievement levels of students in any given classroom.

To their credit, the developers showed the foresight to suggest the need to provide *different* learners, or students with varying entering skills, support services, though their insistence on "mastery level" performances reveals that the developers have a poor understanding of what the term "diversity" truly represents. Notice that

> While the standards set grade-specific goals, they do not define how the standards should be taught or which materials should be used to support students. States and districts recognize that there will need to be a range of supports in place to ensure that all students, including those with special needs and English language learners, can master the standards.[4]

Now we face a potential problem. If Common Core's developers acknowledged that diversity was a potential complication, and that a range of supports would be needed to ensure that all students could *master* the standards, where were these supports to come from? It's one thing to state a need; it's another to deliver. *New York Times* editor, A.H. Weiler (1909–2002), is credited with famously declaring the terse warning "Nothing's impossible to the person who doesn't have to do it." And so again, a group that mentions the importance of an inclusion fails to share with the public how they intend to accomplish that which they believe is necessary. To the group's thorough *discredit*, they opted to play the kindergarten game "Kick the can."

> It is up to the states to define the full range of supports appropriate for these students.[5]

Common Core's overseers passed along the critical obligation to provide student-needed supports to financially strapped states, some with state officials that unabashedly believe that a skeleton crew of teachers is not only enough, it's already an arm and a leg too many. Recall what we learned 25 years ago:

> Being declared eligible for special education [support] services had less to do with the difficulties the child was experiencing with ... school work, and more to do with the state and school district in which the youngster lived.[6]

That doesn't bode well for any of our diverse/different learners who will be expected, along with all their classmates, to arrive at the station on time despite the mile marker from where they started.

Let me be more emphatic. Consider this, please. Two children in the same class, both expected to acquire the same material, one who is a year above grade level in reading and math, and the other who is two years below grade level in reading and math. The children have the same teacher, the same curriculum, and the same Common Core standards. Should we expect that both would arrive on time, at the same time? Most unlikely, is the reasonable reply. The mile marker from which the two start does matter.

You might wonder who wrote the standards?[7] Were Common Core's developers field-tested? Were the authors excellent teachers with a long history of working diligently with the 25 (or more) highly diverse children, each child with his or her own challenging *intra*-subject variability, where the *same* child excels in reading but struggles mightily in math? Did the developers factor in the possibility that some children would need more time than others to master a sequential step, one that's a prerequisite to a subsequent step, like you first need to get to your knees before you crawl before you can walk? The answer might surprise you.

After investigating Common Core, Diane Ravitch, Professor of Education at New York University, discovered that

> The writers of the standards included no early childhood educators, no edu-
> cators of children with disabilities, no experienced classroom teachers;
> indeed, the largest contingent of the drafting committee were *representatives
> of the testing industry*. No attempt was made to have pilot testing of the stan-
> dards in real classrooms with real teachers and students. The standards do not
> permit any means to challenge, correct, or revise them.[8] (Emphasis mine)

The testing industry? That's a strange bedfellow, don't you think? These will be the folks who will make copious, *beaucoup* bucks off the testing arrangement. Many hundreds of millions would be a low guess.[9] Isn't that somewhat like asking the pharmaceutical companies to suggest non-drug options for a child's rowdy classroom behavior? Did no one at the local school level, the state level, or the federal level acknowledge the incredibly diverse children who would be subjected to what the testing industry decided? Were the parents of the children given any voice? Did the US Department of Education stand by and watch the parade go by? Didn't anyone look at the details? Or were the everyday working particulars of this enormous operation soon to impact millions of American school kids dismissed as irrelevant to the larger romantic picture?

> My conversations with several Core proponents over the past few weeks
> leave me with the sense they fell in love with an abstraction and gave barely
> a thought to implementation. But implementation—how a thing is done
> day by day in the real world—is everything.[10] (Peggy Noonan, Reporter, *The
> Wall Street Journal*, May 2014)

CONCERNS

During a web seminar, a classroom teacher raised concern about Common Core and struggling students. Curtis Linton, executive director and co-owner of School Improvement Network, responded: "The Common Core is designed to give teachers flexibility in meeting students' needs—if a student is behind, it is *easy* to go back a few steps and focus on building skills. If a student is ahead of his or her peers, then it is *easy* to move forward and help the student reach the next level according to his or her needs."[11] (Emphases are mine.)

Spoken by someone who by all accounts hasn't ever adjusted Common Core curriculum while managing 25 highly diverse and mostly energetic children. Admiring his many interests and accomplishments, Mr. Linton's bibliography says nothing about him being a classroom teacher. Acknowledging that one doesn't have to jump off a bridge to know that the river below is wet, still, one will need to do more than admire from a safe distance the water's ripples to appreciate its force and unpredictability.)

Some people have spoken out about Common Core, their reactions softened by their penchant to be polite. Consider the following:

"[Any] things about the common core that you don't like?" was asked of Charlotte Danielson, an accepted authority you met in the previous chapter.

Dr. Danielson replied:

I do worry somewhat about the assessments—I'm concerned that we may be headed for a train wreck there. The test items I've seen that have been released so far are extremely challenging. If I had to take a test that was entirely comprised of items like that, I'm not sure that I would pass it—and I've got a bunch of degrees [from Cornell and Oxford Universities]. So I do worry that in some schools we'll have 80 percent or some large number of students failing. That's what I mean by train wreck. But who knows? We just don't know enough about the assessments right now. But when I have shown some of those released items to groups of educators—to teachers and administrators—the room just goes very quiet. So I can imagine a hostile response on the part of some educators and communities. But I'd like to be wrong about that.[12]

That Dr. Danielson admits that she'd "like to be wrong" is a soft admission that she fears she's right.

Once again, what's perceived as current student underachievement has brought us to seek a solution to problems associated with our future social, educational, and economic position in the world. No one likes to read stories that tell of high school graduates with dismal reading and math skills, where even some college-bound students need remedial courses to bring them up to an arbitrary par. A recent Internet video showed random US high school students struggling for answers when asked to "Name a country that starts with the letter 'U'." One student answered, "Europe." When asked to "Name the countries that border the USA," one student begged off saying "There's too many." We're likewise disappointed when we hear that a large percentage of sixth-graders embarrassed themselves and their schools with paltry scores on statewide, standardized science tests. While our collective discontent is noted and appreciated, we're naive if we believe that pasting new curriculum standards on a wall will alone oil the machinery that runs the country's often sputtering graded general education classroom.

> ...The disadvantages of the graded system's rigidity [became] apparent, and by the end of the nineteenth century there were various efforts to create different schooling models and achieve greater flexibility. These efforts continued well into the twentieth century, handicapped to some extent by the publishing industry's success in producing age-graded textbook series that made it easier for teachers to manage their work. In the same period, so-called normal schools and later, colleges, produced teachers whose preparation assumed that each would work alone in a self-contained classroom and, except for those in smaller multi-graded schools, with materials deemed suitable for one age-group of children.[13] (My note. A single age group, or grade level, can have entering skill variability equivalent to 3–4 years. "Children enter the first grade with a range of from three to four years in their readiness to profit from a 'graded minimum essentials' concept of schooling."[14])

Any set of academic standards intended for the entire population of students attending US public schools will produce discrepancies— instances where the newly established standards do not fit all the enrolled children. Common Core provides such a set of standards. If Common Core's standards are fixed, meaning teachers are given little to no leeway to accommodate, problems are inevitable. We've been down that road before where distributions of children on either side of the common curve were affected. In the past, general education dealt with these children poorly. Metaphorically, the poorer got poorer, and the richer got poorer.

Common Core has raised the specter of the past. As you read in Chapter Three, the 1950s were a tumultuous time for parents as they fought against those who blamed their children's curriculum failures on everything but the curriculum standards. Relief came in the form of "Learning Disabilities," a convenient answer that quieted the critics and allowed exhausted parents time to breathe and recapture their confidence. The upside? It forced the hiring of many special education teachers, some with extraordinary talents who immediately extended help to the struggling children. The downside? It allowed general education to wait haplessly for the cavalry to arrive, their mantra being "I don't know how to teach brain-injured children." (Infuriating!) Again, weeks, often months, passed without any assistance offered to the children as special education's wheel of fortune spun, sometimes landing on "eligible" and sometimes missing it. The process is a little better than a crapshoot but not much. Will Common Core's new standards have us repeat this part of history as well? Concerns have been expressed that our previous errors will pale in comparison with what will happen today. No one would benefit from such an outcome.

WORDS

(Anthony Rebora's interview with Dr. Charlotte Danielson.)[15]

Q: How will the common core affect teachers who have students with a wide range of skill levels or high needs?

A: That is the perennial instructional challenge—kids come into your classroom with a huge range of backgrounds and skills. I fear that the common core papers over that problem.

Q: In what way?

Well, in mathematics, for example, you're expected to focus on a few key concepts for 3rd graders. But suppose you've got some students who never mastered the 1st grade skills. The standards documentation, as far as I can see, is silent on how a teacher handles that situation. ... Say I'm a 4th grade teacher and prime numbers is a 4th grade skill, but I've got some 4th graders who don't understand place value. In that case, my own personal inclination would be to ensure that my students develop conceptual understanding of place value at that point—because that's what they need. ... I don't see how you can responsibly say anything other than that you have to be flexible and teach students what they have the background to learn at that point. Otherwise, you're setting them up for failure.

(Elizabeth Farrell, Scholastic). In the furious national debate over the Common Core standards, there has been little talk of how to accommodate ELL [English Language Learners] and special education students. Yet if you ask educators who work with these kids, you'll hear an equal mix of optimism and concern. Depending on how the standards are applied, they say, implementation could bring unprecedented improvement or unparalleled failure.[16]

(Catherine Gewertz. Education Week. October 2013. A Common-Core Challenge: Learners with Special Needs). Designing...lessons for the typical student is tough enough for teachers; adapting them to children at wildly varied points on the skills spectrum is tougher still. Meeting the needs of students with disabilities, those learning English, those from disadvantaged backgrounds, and gifted students is a challenge that goes to the core of education's purpose, however. And it's a challenge that is largely unmet, more than two years after every state but four adopted [Common Core's] standards.[17]

(Diane Ravitch. Blog. February, 2013. "Why I Cannot Support the Common Core Standards.")... Another reason I cannot support the Common Core standards is that I am worried that they will cause a precipitous decline in test scores, based on arbitrary cut scores, and this will have a disparate impact on students who are English language learners, students with disabilities, and students who are poor and low-performing. A principal in the Mid-West told me that his school piloted the Common Core assessments and the failure rate rocketed upwards, especially among the students with the highest needs....[18]

(Katharine Beals. *The Atlantic*. "The Common Core Is Tough on Kids with Special Needs: The standards don't allow enough flexibility for students who learn differently.")... Restricting students to curricula beyond their [present readiness] substantially lowers their achievement. Success for all requires openness towards cognitive diversity....[19]

Discussing testing results and their implications, Janet Roberts, Director of Education and Director of Product Development of Aristotle Circle, commented: Almost half of the New York City's students were failing the old tests that were considered less difficult to pass [than Common Core's tests]. ... [S]ummer school may only be available for kids who fail miserably. ... In order to keep summer school attendance from skyrocketing, some students may be allowed to fail their high stakes exams and get to move on without learning the skills required of their grade or needed to prepare for success in the next grade. This latest change may mean that students who fail may be ... left to fill in the gaps on their own without any additional educational support to bring them up to grade-level.

How ironic. With school being for many the only chance to make something of themselves, we pull that safety net out from under their inevitable fall. Whether tutoring can bolster enough is to be seen.[20]

RIGID STANDARDS, DIVERSE STUDENTS

Common Core's standards set grade-specific goals.[21] The standards specify what skills and content a child *should* know at a given point in time. This absence of flexibility is intentional. On paper, the skills a third-grader in Florida is expected to learn are the same as the skills a third-grader in Iowa is expected to learn. However, we learned that

[w]hile the standards set grade-specific goals, they do not define how the standards should be taught or which materials should be used to support students. States and districts recognize that there will need to be a range of supports in place to ensure that all students, including those with special needs and English language learners, can master the standards.[22]

In other words, schools, teachers, and districts can teach the specifics as they choose. Some schools and some teachers will do a much better job educating children than others. The lack of consistent results among our public schools comes as no surprise. But with Common Core, the problem takes a decidedly more serious turn. We're not talking about individual classroom teachers developing their own tests based entirely on what they have taught their children, what we can call "criterion-referenced" tests that test the criteria that were presented to the children. Not with Common Core. The assessment process that ultimately grades our school children as passing and/or failing relies on one publisher's test, a publisher with no need to concern itself with students who are diverse/different/ exceptional learners, a publisher who doesn't need to concern itself with any *health* effects its instrument may have on our kids.

It's almost midnight, and my daughter is calling to me. She went to bed hours ago, but she is so stressed—at age 10—that she can't sleep. She will do this nearly every night for two weeks until she finally takes the long-dreaded ... State English Language Arts exam. Pearson [Publishers] is a palpable presence in her education. ... The company developed much of the school's fourth-grade English curriculum as part of the Common Core standards. Pearson also designed the test for it. All of this in an education world where tests increasingly are the be-all and end-all. "Mom," she says, tears spilling onto her pillow, "why is one test so important?" She answers her own question with grim, distressing logic: "If I don't do well on the fourth-grade test, I won't get into a good middle school. If I don't get into a good middle school, then I won't get into a good high school, and if I don't do that, I won't get into a good college, and then I won't get a good job." I cringe, feeling that I have failed as a parent if this is what she believes. And yet she has a point. [T]hat ... test helps determine which middle school you get into. In her classroom, the pressure was so great that the teacher referred to the tests by aliases: the "waka-waka" and the "whablah." They were the elementary-school equivalent, it seemed, of Harry Potter's nemesis Voldemort, more commonly referred to as "he who must not be named."[23]

"[D]octors increasingly see children in early elementary school suffering from migraine headaches and ulcers. Many physicians see a clear connection to performance pressure. 'I'm talking about 5-, 6-, 7-year-olds who are coming in with these conditions. We never used to see that,' says Lawrence Rosen, a New Jersey pediatrician who works with pediatric associations nationally. 'I'm hearing this from my colleagues everywhere.'"[24]

The question must be asked: What are we doing in the name of education?

Parents need to see relief in the classroom from inappropriate standards. The tests need to be diagnostic and helpful for children. ... [T]est and punish must end.[25] (Lisa Rudley, New York Allies for Public Education)

(FYI: More than 100 university-based education researchers in California called for a moratorium on Common Core testing. Overall, there is not a compelling body of research supporting the notion that a nationwide set of curriculum standards, including those like the CCSS [Common Core State Standards], will either raise the quality of education for all children or close the gap between different groups of children. In spring 2015, 3.2 million students in California (grades 3-8 and 11) took the new, computerized Math and English Language Arts/Literacy ... tests. Scores were released to the public in September 2015, and as many predicted, a majority of students failed, that is, were categorized to be below proficient).[26] (Diane Ravitch, April 9, 2016)

Common core will produce curriculum requirements that are well-beyond many children's readiness skills. Unavoidably, the children will struggle, as will their concerned parents. Through no fault of their own, the children will be prime targets for the medical model, with the favored disabilities, ADHD and LD, poised as explanations for the children's curriculum difficulties.

Our responsibility to the children demands that we recognize the culprit is not a biological flaw within the child, but a presumptuous educational system that once again has thought more about its standards and itself than its diverse pupils and their singular needs. We must see each child as an individual with his/her own entering skills, not as a member of a collective group that shares age, grade level, and the same curriculum, not if we care about the children.

NOTES

1. Preparing American students for success. (2017). *corestandards.org*. Retrieved from http://www.corestandards.org.
2. Heitner, E. (2013). The trouble with common core. *rethinkingschools.org*. Retrieved from http://www.rethinkingschools.org/archive/27_04/edit274.shtml.
3. Standards in your state. (2017). *corestandards.org*. Retrieved from http://www.corestandards.org/standards-in-your-state/.
4. Preparing American students for success. (2017).
5. Read the standards. (2017). *corestandards.org*. Retrieved from http://www.corestandards.org/read-the-standards/.
6. Reynolds, C.R. (1990). Conceptual and technical problems in learning disability diagnosis. In C.R. Reynolds & R.W. Kamphaus, (Eds.), *Handbook of psychological and educational assessment of children: Intelligence and achievement* (p. 574). New York: Guilford.
7. Who wrote the common core standards? The common core 24. (n.d.) *seattleducation2010.wordpress.com*. Retrieved from https://seattleducation2010.wordpress.com/common-core-standards/who-wrote-the-common-core-standards-the-common-core-24/.
8. Dardick, F. (June 28, 2014). Bill Gates' Reckless Meddling With U.S. Education Through Common Core. *redstate.com*. Retrieved from http://www.redstate.com/diary/fdardick/2014/06/18/bill-gates-reckless-meddling-u-s-education-common-core/.
9. Strauss, V. (September 23, 2015). Common Core: 'the gift that Pearson counts on to keep giving'. *washingtonpost.com*. Retrieved from https://www.washingtonpost.com/news/answer-sheet/wp/2015/09/23/com-

mon-core-the-gift-that-pearson-counts-on-to-keep-giving/?utm_term=.
cbf925fd1d64.

10. Noonan, P. (May 7, 2014). The Trouble with Common Core. *blog.wsj.
com*. Retrieved from http://blogs.wsj.com/peggynoonan/2014/05/07/
the-trouble-with-common-core/.

11. Heath, J. (November 4, 2011). Common core designed to give teachers
flexibility, says Curtis Linton. *schoolimprovement.com*. Retrieved from
http://www.schoolimprovement.com/common-core-360/blog/
Common-Core-Designed-to-Give-Teachers-Flexibility-Says-Curtis-
Linton/.

12. Pipkin, C. (2014). Charlotte Danielson on Teaching and the Common
Core. See: http://www.schoolimprovement.com/common-core-360/
blog/common-core-standards-charlotte-danielson/.

13. http://education.stateuniversity.com/pages/2297/ Nongraded-Schools.
html.

14. Goodlad and Anderson, p. 27 Goodlad, J.I., & Anderson, R.H. (1987). The
nongraded elementary school. (p. 27). New York: Teacher's College Press.

15. Pipkin, C. (2014).

16. Farrell, E. (2013). Adapting the core. *scholastic.com*. Retrieved from
http://www.scholastic.com/browse/article.jsp?id=3758233.

17. Gewertz, C. A Common-Core Challenge: Learners with Special Needs:
Adapting the standards for students with disabilities, English-learners, and
gifted students is no easy task. *edweek.org*. Retrieved from http://www.
edweek.org/ew/articles/2013/10/30/10cc-intro.h33.html.

18. Ravitch, D. (February 26, 2013). Why I cannot support the common core
standards. *dianeravitch.net*. Retrieved from http://dianeravitch.
net/2013/02/26/why-i-cannot-support-the-common-core-standards/.

19. Beals, K. (February 21, 2014). The Common Core Is Tough on
Kids with Special Needs. The standards don't allow enough flexibility for students who learn differently. *theatlantic.com*. Retrieved
from http://www.theatlantic.com/education/archive/2014/02/
the-common-core-is-tough-on-kids-with-special-needs/283973/.

20. Glum, J. (March 3, 2013). Common Core Tutoring Companies See
Business Boom Ahead of Spring Tests As Parents, Students Struggle With
Standards. *ibtimes.com*. Retrieved from http://www.ibtimes.com/
common-core-tutoring-companies-see-business-boom-ahead-spring-
tests-parents-students-1834784.

21. Read the standards. (2017).

22. Preparing American students for success. (2017).

23. Reingold, J. (2015). Everybody hates Pearson. *fortune.com*. Retrieved
from http://fortune.com/2015/01/21/everybody-hates-pearson/.

24. Abeles, Vicki. (January 2, 2016). Is the drive for success making our
children sick? *nytimes.com*. Retrieved from https://www.nytimes.

com/2016/01/03/opinion/sunday/is-the-drive-for-success-making-our-children-sick.html.

25. Strauss, V. (April 2, 2016). How many students are refusing to take common core tests this year. *washingtonpost.com*. https://www.washingtonpost.com/news/answer-sheet/wp/2016/04/06/how-many-students-are-refusing-to-take-common-core-tests-this-year/.

26. Moore, N.R. (April 9, 2016). More than 100 California researchers call for a moratorium on common core assessments. *novemoore.wordpress.com*. Retrieved from https://novemoore.wordpress.com/2016/04/09/more-than-100-california-researchers-call-for-moratorium-on-common-core-assessments/.

INDEX

eligibility determinations and, 35, 39, 48, 49, 53
experience quotient and, 43, 46
general education revenues, encroachment on, 37
heterogeneous groups of children and, 56
identification/measurement of, 35, 37, 38, 41, 47, 48, 52, 53, 71
innate intelligence and, 40–43, 45
intelligence, flawed definition/ measurement of, 42
intelligence tests, narrow measurement potential of, 43–45
intervention blueprints and, 54
IQ-Achievement Discrepancy Model and, 40–42, 47
LD movement and, 34
"learning disabilities" term, origin of, 38, 48, 56
learning disability benchmark and, 40
litigious environment and, 39
medical model explanation of, 52, 59, 61, 68
medical profession, interest of, 34
minimal brain dysfunction syndrome and, 65
multidisciplinary team diagnosis of, 49
non-learning disability benchmark and, 40
noun phrase "learning disability disorder" and, 65
parent involvement, advocacy role and, 31–34, 39
pint jug metaphor, educable capacity and, 44
prevalence of, 34–35
prevention/remediation orientation and, 52

referrals for services, excessive number of, 29
research-based interventions and, 53–55
response to intervention/multi-tiered system of supports and, 51–54
specific learning disability category and, 33, 48
"uneducable" students, historic exclusion of, 29
valid measurement standards, lack of, 42
See also Active intervention; Attention deficit/hyperactivity disorder (ADHD); Disability identification; Intelligence; Intelligence quotient (IQ) tests; Underachievement
Least restrictive environment (LRE), 8
Lejeune, Jérôme, 136
Linton, Curtis, 226

M
Martin, Reed, 29
Mechanic, David, 109
Medical model, 18
  attention deficit/hyperactivity disorder and, 97, 105, 109, 110, 153, 168, 169, 173–176, 182, 183
  Down syndrome and, 136
  learning disabilities and, 52, 59, 61, 62, 64, 70, 71
Melchior, Maria, 91, 139
Merrow, John, 183
Minimal brain dysfunction syndrome (MBDS), 64, 65, 114
  See also Attention deficit/ hyperactivity disorder (ADHD); Disability identification; Learning disabilities

Sputnik launch, 20
Standards movement, 19, 22
See also Common Core Standards
(CCSS)
State-run facility, *see* Behavioral
psychology laboratory
Sternberg, Robert, 48
Survival anxiety, 20
Szasz, Thomas, 89

T
Tautologies, 144, 228
Thapar, Anita, 120
Thoner, Sharon, 205
Torgesen, Joe, 52
Trisomy 21, 136, 138

U
Underachievement
Cold War education scare and,
20–21
deficit perspective and, 10–11
education's germ theory and, 18,
23, 34
failing school systems and, 16, 21
institutionalization/medicalization
of, 10, 11, 59
labeling practices and, 9
learning disability programs and, 16
regular education students vs.
severely involved population
and, 11

special services referrals, rationales
for, 11–12
standard teaching practices and, 11
standards movement and, 19
"Uneducable" students, 29–30
University of Denver, *see* Cooperative
school; Educational practices

V
van Pragg, Herman, 162

W
Walker, Sidney, III, 174
Waring, Dana, 134
Wechsler, David, 43, 207
Wechsler Intelligence Test for Children
(WISC), 41
Weiler, Abe H., 224
Wender, Paul, 117
Whalen, Carol, 179
Wheldall, Kevin, 211
Whitaker, Robert, 178
Willcut, Erik, 120
Willerman, Lee, 129
Wilson, Sloan, 21
Wood, Alexis, 132
Woodcock-Johnson Achievement
Test, 41

Z
Zeidner, Daniel L., 216